Clinical Cases in
Endodontics

Clinical Cases Series

Wiley-Blackwell's Clinical Cases series is designed to recognize the centrality of clinical cases to the dental profession by providing actual cases with an academic backbone. This unique approach supports the new trend in case-based and problem-based learning. Highly illustrated in full color, the Clinical Cases series utilizes a format that fosters independent learning and prepares the reader for case-based examinations.

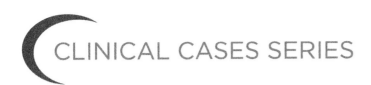

CLINICAL CASES SERIES

Clinical Cases in
Endodontics

Takashi Komabayashi
University of New England

WILEY Blackwell

Registered Office
John Wiley & Sons, Inc., 111 River Street, Hoboken, NJ 07030, USA

Editorial Office
111 River Street, Hoboken, NJ 07030, USA

For details of our global editorial offices, customer services, and more information about Wiley products visit us at www.wiley.com.

Wiley also publishes its books in a variety of electronic formats and by print-on-demand. Some content that appears in standard print versions of this book may not be available in other formats.

Library of Congress Cataloging-in-Publication Data

Names: Komabayashi, Takashi, 1973- editor.
Title: Clinical cases in endodontics / edited by Takashi Komabayashi.
Description: Hoboken, NJ : Wiley, 2017. | Series: Clinical cases series |
   Includes bibliographical references and index. |
Identifiers: LCCN 2017020926 (print) | LCCN 2017021343 (ebook) | ISBN
   9781119147114 (pdf) | ISBN 9781119147060 (epub) | ISBN 9781119147046 (pbk.)
Subjects: | MESH: Root Canal Therapy–methods | Endodontics–methods | Case
   Reports
Classification: LCC RK351 (ebook) | LCC RK351 (print) | NLM WU 230 | DDC
   617.6/342–dc23
LC record available at https://lccn.loc.gov/2017020926

Cover Design: Wiley
Cover Images: (Column 1) Courtesy of Howard Foo;(Column 2) Courtesy of Qiang Zhu and Keivan
              Zoufan;(Column 3) Courtesy of Nathaniel Nicholson

Set in 10/13pt Univers LTStd by SPi Global, Chennai, India

10 9 8 7 6 5 4 3 2 1

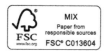

CONTENTS

CONTENTS

CONTRIBUTORS

Editor

Takashi Komabayashi, DDS, MDS, PhD, Diplomate, American Board of Endodontics, Clinical Professor, University of New England College of Dental Medicine, Portland, Maine, USA.

Chapter Authors

Jeffrey Albert, DMD, Diplomate, American Board of Endodontics, Private Practice, Endodontic Associates, West Palm Beach, Florida, USA.

Abdullah Alqaied, DDS, MDS, Diplomate, American Board of Endodontics, Private Practice, Asnan Tower, Al-Salmiya, Kuwait.

Bruce Y. Cha, DMD, FAGD, FACD, FICD, Diplomate, American Board of Endodontics, Private Practice, Endodontic LLC, New Haven and Hamden; Section Chief, Endodontics, Department of Dentistry, Yale-New Haven Hospital, New Haven; Assistant Clinical Professor, Yale School of Medicine, New Haven; Assistant Clinical Professor, Division of Endodontology, School of Dental Medicine, University of Connecticut, Farmington, Connecticut, USA.

Priya S. Chand, BDS, MSD, Diplomate, American Board of Endodontics, Clinical Associate Professor, Division of Endodontics, University of Maryland Dental School, Baltimore, Maryland, USA.

Daniel Chavarría-Bolaños, DDS, MSc, PhD, Professor/Researcher, Facultad de Odontología, Universidad de Costa Rica, San José, Costa Rica.

Kana Chisaka-Miyara, DDS, PhD, Part-time Lecturer, Department of Pulp Biology and Endodontics, Tokyo Medical and Dental University, Tokyo, Japan.

Suanhow Howard Foo, DDS, Diplomate, American Board of Endodontics, Private Practice, Hacienda Heights, California, USA.

Denise Foran, DDS, Diplomate, American Board of Endodontics, Program Director/Advanced Specialty Program in Endodontics, Department of Veterans Affairs New York Harbor Healthcare System, New York, USA.

Nada Ibrahim, BDS, Saudi Board of Endodontics, University Staff Clinics, College of Dentistry, King Saud University, Riyadh, Saudi Arabia.

Ahmed O Jamleh, BDS, MSc., PhD, Assistant Professor of Endodontics, Restorative and Prosthetic Dental Sciences, College of Dentistry, King Saud bin Abdulaziz University for Health Sciences, National Guard Health Affairs, Riyadh, Saudi Arabia.

Jin Jiang, DDS, PhD, Diplomate, American Board of Endodontics, Private Practice, Endodontic LLC, New Haven and Hamden; Assistant Professor, Division of Endodontology, University of Connecticut School of Dental Medicine, Farmington, Connecticut, USA.

Bill Kahler, DClinDent, PhD, School of Dentistry, University of Queensland, Brisbane, Australia.

Takashi Komabayashi, DDS, MDS, PhD, Diplomate, American Board of Endodontics, Clinical Professor, University of New England College of Dental Medicine, Portland, Maine, USA.

Louis M. Lin, BDS, DMD, PhD, Diplomate, American Board of Endodontics, Professor, Department of Endodontics, New York University College of Dentistry, New York, USA.

David Masuoka-Ito, DDS, PhD, Researcher Professor, Department of Somatology, Universidad Autónoma de Aguascalientes, Aguascalientes, México.

Katia Mattos, DMD, Diplomate, American Board of Endodontics, Private Practice, Miami, Florida, USA.

Nathaniel T. Nicholson, DDS, MS, Diplomate, American Board of Endodontics, Private Practice, Galesville, MD; Clinical Assistant Professor, West Virginia University School of Dentistry, Morgantown, West Virginia, USA.

Takashi Okiji, DDS, PhD, Professor, Department of Pulp Biology and Endodontics, Graduate School of Medical and Dental Sciences, Tokyo Medical and Dental University, Tokyo, Japan.

Pejman Parsa, DDS, MS, Diplomate, American Board of Endodontics, Private Practice, West LA Endodontics, Los Angeles, California, USA.

Amaury J. Pozos-Guillén, DDS, MSc, PhD, Professor, Facultad de Estomatología, Universidad Autónoma de San Luis Potosí, San Luis Potosí, SLP, México.

Amr Radwan, BDS, Diplomate, American Board of Endodontics, Private Practice, Miami, Florida, USA.

Jessica Russo Revand, DMD, MS, Private Practice, Northern Virginia Endodontic Associates, Arlington, Virginia, USA.

John M. Russo, DMD, Associate Clinical Professor, Division of Endodontics, University of Connecticut School of Dental Medicine, Farmington, Connecticut, USA.

Khaled Seifelnasr, BDS, DDS, MS, Private Practice, Hudson, New Hampshire; Lecturer on Restorative Dentistry and Biomaterials Sciences, Harvard School of Dental Medicine, Boston, Massachusetts, USA.

Andrew L. Shur, DMD, Diplomate, American Board of Endodontics, Private Practice, Endodontic Associates, Portland, Assistant Clinical Professor, University of New England College of Dental Medicine, Portland, Maine, USA.

Savita Singh, DDS, Private Practice, New York, USA.

Victoria E. Tountas, DDS, Diplomate, American Board of Endodontics, Private Practice, Plano, Texas, USA.

Gayatri Vohra, DDS, Private Practice, Acton and Concord Endodontics, Lecturer on Restorative Dentistry and Biomaterials Sciences, Harvard School of Dental Medicine, Boston, Massachusetts, USA.

Andrew Xu, DDS, MS, Diplomate, American Board of Endodontics, Private Practice, Plano, Texas, USA.

Yoshio Yahata, DDS, PhD, Assistant Professor, Division of Endodontology, Department of Conservative Dentistry, Showa University School of Dentistry, Tokyo, Japan.

Maobin Yang, DMD, MDS, PhD, Diplomate, American Board of Endodontics, Assistant Professor, Department of Endodontology, Kornberg School of Dentistry, Temple University, Philadelphia, Pennsylvania, USA.

Parisa Zakizadeh, DDS, MS, Diplomate, American Board of Endodontics, Private Practice, La Jolla Dental Specialty Group, San Diego, California, USA.

Qiang Zhu, DDS, PhD, Diplomate, American Board of Endodontics, Professor, Division of Endodontology, University of Connecticut School of Dental Medicine, Farmington, Connecticut, USA.

Keivan Zoufan, DDS, MDS, Diplomate, American Board of Endodontics, Private Practice, Zoufan Endodontics, Los Altos and Cupertino, Assistant Professor of Dental Diagnostic Science, University of the Pacific, Arthur A. Dugoni School of Dentistry, San Francisco, California, USA.

ACKNOWLEDGEMENTS

The editor and contributors would like to acknowledge the great help they have received from colleagues and students.

Special support came from:

Elizabeth J. Dyer, MLIS, AHIP (Associate Dean of Library Services, Research & Teaching Librarian, University of New England); **Miki Furusho** PhD (Image analysis consultant, University of Connecticut); **Kathy Hooke**, MAT, JD (English language consultant); **Christine Lin** (Assistant); **Oran Suta** (Medical/Dental illustration, University of New England College of Osteopathic Medicine).

The following students at the University of New England College of Dental Medicine reviewed and provided invaluable feedback on this textbook:

Brittney Bell, Aparna Bhat, Dorothy Cataldo, Hannah Chung, Lindsey Cunningham, Sarah Georgeson, Andy Greenslade, Keith Hau, Anna Ivanova, Alex Katanov, Jonathan Nutt, Tara Prasad, Rishi Phakey, Christine Roenitz, Tarandeep Sidiura, Arina Sorokina, Shadbeh Taghizadeh, Eleanor Threet, Jackson Threet, Anh Tran, Robert Walsh, Minjin Yoo, Kenneth Yuth.

Professional clinical input and critical reviews were generously provided by the following valued colleagues (endodontists, endo residents and periodontists):

Anthony J. Carter, DDS, Advanced Specialty Program in Endodontics/Resident (Class of 2017), Department of Veterans Affairs New York Harbor Healthcare System, New York, USA.

Akira Hasuike, DDS, PhD, Assistant Professor, Nihon University School of Dentistry, Tokyo, Japan.

Rachel McKee Garoufalis, DMD, Private Practice, Manchester, New Hampshire; Assistant Clinical Professor, University of New England College of Dental Medicine, Portland, Maine, USA.

Rick Moser, DDS, Advanced Specialty Program in Endodontics/Resident (Class of 2016), Department of Veterans Affairs New York Harbor Healthcare System, New York, USA.

Lester Reid, DMD, MDS, Private Practice, Hartford, Assistant Clinical Professor, University of Connecticut Health Center, Farmington, Connecticut, USA.

Manuel Sato, DDS, Advanced Specialty Program in Endodontics/Resident (Class of 2020), University of Connecticut Health Center, Farmington, Connecticut, USA.

Chase Thompson, DMD, Advanced Specialty Program in Endodontics/Resident (Class of 2018), Department of Veterans Affairs New York Harbor Healthcare System, New York, USA.

1

Introduction

Takashi Komabayashi

LEARNING OBJECTIVES
- To understand the purpose, special features, and benefits of this book.
- To understand the scope and approach of each chapter.
- To understand the terminology and common frames of reference used.

Copiously illustrated in full color, *Clinical Cases in Endodontics* brings together actual endodontic clinical cases chosen by national and international master clinicians and leading academics, building from the simple to the complex and from the common to the rare. Part of the Wiley-Blackwell Clinical Cases series, and with cases ranging from nonsurgical root canal treatment to complicated therapy, this book presents practical, everyday applications accompanied by rigorously supported academic commentary in a unique approach that questions and educates readers about essential topics in clinical endodontics. The format of *Clinical Cases in Endodontics* fosters case-based, problem-based and evidence-based independent learning and prepares readers for case-based examinations. It is, therefore, useful as a textbook from which predoctoral dental students and postgraduate residents may learn about the challenging and absorbing nature of endodontic treatment. However, the book's range and depth of detail will also make it an excellent reference tool for practitioners whenever perplexing cases arise in the dental office.

Each chapter provides a brief recap of key theoretical concepts, situates cases within the framework of standard protocols, and considers the advantages and disadvantages of the clinical regimen. This approach enables student readers to build their skills, aiding their ability to think critically and independently. However, by simulating a step-by-step visual presentation, this book also facilitates development and refinement of technique regardless of one's years of experience in endodontic treatment. *Clinical Cases in Endodontics* will make all readers more confident in their understanding of endodontic treatment.

Composition of each Chapter (Chapters 2 to 25)
Clinical Cases in Endodontics adheres to the same four-part structure for each chapter.

1. Learning Objectives
Each chapter opens with a statement of learning objectives for that chapter, a format familiar from course syllabi at many dental schools or dental continuing education courses.

2. Clinical Case (With Radiographs and Pictures)
The focus of each chapter is a single case, presented in the case-based format of the American Board of Endodontics (ABE) Case History Exam. Since this book is intended for dental students and general dentists, as well as endodontic residents and endodontic specialists, the level of case difficulty may not be the same as that reflected in the ABE Case History Exam. All cases are real cases, however, chosen by master

clinicians and/or leading academics for uniqueness and complexity. Overall, the level of difficulty is high.

The following are common guidelines used by all authors for each chapter.

- The dental notation system in this textbook is the "Universal Tooth Designation System" used in the United States (i.e., tooth #1 to #32). If you are a student/resident/dentist outside the United States, it is likely that your country/region is using a different tooth designation system, such as the International Standards Organization designation system (ISO System) by Fédération Dentaire Internationale (FDI) World Dental Federation or Palmer method. International readers may consult Figure 1.1 to see how these systems relate to one another. International coverage and perspectives will be sought. The Pulpal & Apical Diagnostic Terminology (Figure 1.2) used in this textbook follows that published in the December 2009 special issue of the *Journal of Endodontics*. Also consulted were *Mosby's Dental Dictionary* (Mosby 2013) and *Dentistry at a Glance* (Kay 2016).
- In each chapter, text, radiographs and pictures, including many follow-up radiographs and clinical photos, combine to provide sufficient and necessary detail for understanding each case. Taken together, the individual cases demonstrate the full scope of the field of endodontics.
- Unlike other endodontics textbooks, each chapter provides a detailed history, diagnosis, and treatment procedures for the case described. The case series focuses on using critical thinking and analysis to merge concepts and actual patient treatments.
- *Clinical Cases in Endodontics* uses a case- and evidence-based format throughout, with appropriate citations and references.

Structure of clinical cases
- Chief Complaint
- Medical History
- Dental History
- Clinical Evaluation (Diagnostic Procedures)
  - Examinations (Extra-oral and Intra-oral)
  - Diagnostic Tests (Summarized in Table)
  - Radiographic Findings
- Pretreatment Diagnosis
  - Pulpal
  - Apical
- Treatment Plan
  - Recommended
  - Alternative

- Restorative
- Prognosis (Favorable, Questionable, or Unfavorable)
- Clinical Procedures: Treatment Record
- Post-Treatment Evaluation

3. Five Self-Study Questions
The self-study questions will be useful at all levels to assess mastery of the concepts and techniques set forth in the chapter. A student might use them in studying for midterm and final exams at a dental school or residency program, an endodontic resident might use them to prepare for a mock oral examination, or an endodontist to prepare for board examinations. The self-study questions may also serve as an abstract and publications writing tool for endodontic professionals.

4. Answers to the Five Self-Study Questions (With References)
A full answer is provided for each self-study question, backed up by references to peer-reviewed publications (original articles and review articles).

Benefits of this book
Clinical Cases in Endodontics is not just another "how you do things" textbook. Nor is it simply a series of "good-looking root canals." In addition to the stimulus of a step-by-step visual (photographic) presentation, similar to the ABE examinations, explanations of treatment modality and clinical background are supported by contemporary, evidence-based research. Cases include the whole scope of endodontics treatment, including medical and dental history, examination and diagnosis, treatments, and outcome assessments. The unique combination of breadth and depth gives rise to numerous benefits for a wide range of dental students, residents and endodontic practitioners. The book:
- supports analysis of problem etiology and application of critical thinking;
- fosters comparison and evaluation of alternative approaches, with rationales for plans of action and predicted outcomes;
- creates a simulation-type environment in which students/residents/dentists may engage in decision-making;
- allows for retrospective critiques of cases to identify error and its causes, as well as recognition of exemplary performance;
- encourages analysis and discussion of students'/ residents'/ dentists' work products in comparison

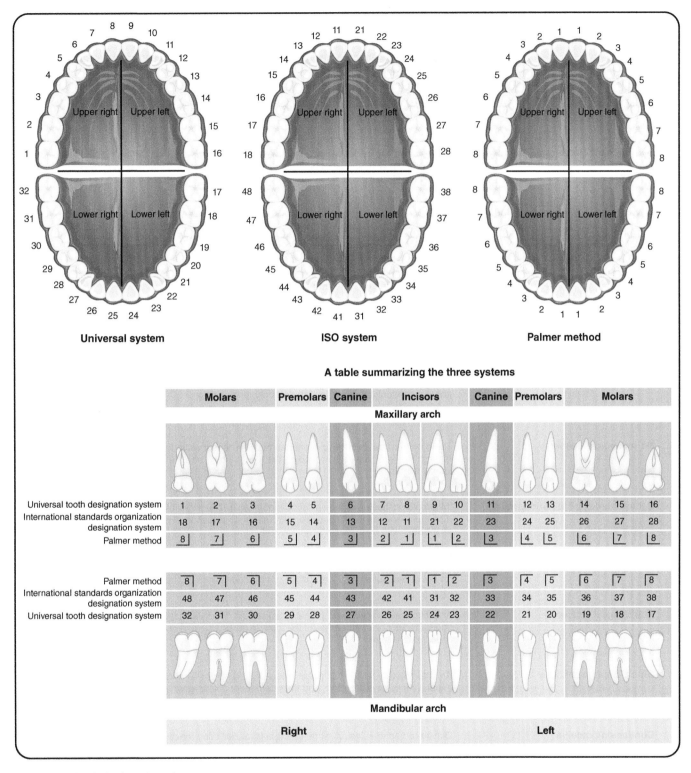

Figure 1.1 Tooth designation: three system summary.

with best-evidence outcomes or other professional standards;
- encourages active learning methods, such as case analysis and discussion, critical appraisal of scientific

evidence in combination with clinical application and patient factors; and structured sessions in which students/ residents/ dentists reason aloud about patient care.

Pulpal:

Normal pulp	A clinical diagnostic category in which the pulp is symptom-free and normally responsive to pulp testing.
Reversible pulpitis	A clinical diagnosis based upon subjective and objective findings indicating that the inflammation should resolve and the pulp return to normal.
Symptomatic irreversible pulpitis	A clinical diagnosis based on subjective and objective findings indicating that the vital inflamed pulp is incapable of healing. *Additional descriptors*: Lingering thermal pain, spontaneous pain, referred pain.
Asymptomatic irreversible pulpitis	A clinical diagnosis based on subjective and objective findings indicating that the vital inflamed pulp is incapable of healing. *Additional descriptors*: No clinical symptoms but inflammation produced by caries, caries excavation, trauma.
Pulp necrosis	A clinical diagnostic category indicating death of the dental pulp. The pulp is usually non-responsive to pulp testing.
Previously treated	A clinical diagnostic category indicating that the tooth has been endodontically treated and the canals are obturated with various filling materials other than intracanal medicaments.
Previously initiated therapy	A clinical diagnostic category indicating that the tooth has been previously treated by partial endodontic therapy (e.g., pulpotomy, pulpectomy).

Apical:

Normal apical tissues	Teeth with normal periradicular tissues that are not sensitive to percussion or palpation testing. The lamina dura surrounding the root is intact, and the periodontal ligament space is uniform.
Symptomatic apical periodontitis	Inflammation, usually of the apical periodontium, producing clinical symptoms including a painful response to biting and/or percussion or palpation. It might or might not be associated with an apical radiolucent area.
Asymptomatic apical periodontitis	Inflammation and destruction of apical periodontium that is of pulpal origin, appears as an apical radiolucent area, and does not produce clinical symptoms.
Acute apical abscess	An inflammatory reaction to pulpal infection and necrosis characterized by rapid onset, spontaneous pain, tenderness of the tooth to pressure, pus formation, and swelling of associated tissues.
Chronic apical abscess	An inflammatory reaction to pulpal infection and necrosis characterized by gradual onset, little or no discomfort, and the intermittent discharge of pus through an associated sinus tract.
Condensing osteitis	Diffuse radiopaque lesion representing a localized bony reaction to a low-grade inflammatory stimulus, usually seen at apex of tooth.

Figure 1.2 Pulpal and apical diagnostic terminology.

References

AAE consensus conference recommended diagnostic terminology. (2009) *Journal of Endodontics* **35**, 1634.

Mosby (2013) *Mosby's Dental Dictionary*, 3rd edn. Amsterdam: Elsevier.

Kay, E. (2016) *Dentistry at a Glance*. Oxford: Wiley–Blackwell.

2

Diagnostic Case I:
Tooth Fracture: Unrestorable

Suanhow Howard Foo

LEARNING OBJECTIVES
- To apply knowledge of dental anatomy to clinical procedures involving a cracked tooth.
- To be able to interpret radiographs used in endodontic diagnosis.
- To formulate a correct endodontic diagnosis and treatment plan based on a variety of clinical testing procedures, taking into account factors such as loss of tooth structure, bruxism, age, and gender.
- To understand the prognosis and incidence rates of the various types of root fractures.

	Molars			Premolars		Canine	Incisors				Canine	Premolars		Molars		
	Maxillary arch															
Universal tooth designation system	1	2	3	4	5	6	7	8	9	10	11	12	13	14	15	16
International standards organization designation system	18	17	16	15	14	13	12	11	21	22	23	24	25	26	27	28
Palmer method	8	7	6	5	4	3	2	1	1	2	3	4	5	6	7	8
Palmer method	8	7	6	5	4	3	2	1	1	2	3	4	5	6	7	8
International standards organization designation system	48	47	46	45	44	43	42	41	31	32	33	34	35	36	37	38
Universal tooth designation system	32	31	30	29	28	27	26	25	24	23	22	21	20	19	18	17
	Mandibular arch															
	Right								**Left**							

Clinical Cases in Endodontics, First Edition. Edited by Takashi Komabayashi.
© 2018 John Wiley & Sons, Inc. Published 2018 by John Wiley & Sons, Inc.

Chief Complaint

"I had excruciating pain last night, now I can't touch my tooth."

Medical History

The patient (Pt) was a 58-year-old male Caucasian. He presented with nothing significant in medical history and no allergies to any medications or to latex. Vital signs were: Blood pressure (BP) 132/87 mmHg, pulse 82 beats per minute (BPM), respiratory rate (RR) 17 breaths per minute.

The Pt was American Society of Anesthesiologists Physical Status Scale (ASA) Class II.

Dental History

Pt had on-and-off pain on the lower right quadrant for a few weeks and was referred for an evaluation of tooth #31. The tooth had a mesial (M) to distal (D) crack. The tooth was painful to touch and the Pt could not eat or bite on that tooth. Pt reported a history of bruxism.

Clinical Evaluation (Diagnostic Procedures)
Examinations
Extra-oral Examination (EOE)

No asymmetry, no lymphadenopathy, no deviation of jaw when opening, no swelling, and temporomandibular joint (TMJ) was within normal limits (WNL).

Intra-oral examination (IOE)

Oral cancer screening performed with all tissues WNL. Tooth #31 had a M to D crack. Periodontal exam showed probing depths from M to D of Facial (4 mm, 3 mm and 8 mm) and M to D of Lingual (4 mm, 4 mm and 8 mm). Tooth #31 had type 1 mobility. Tooth #30 had probing depths from M to D of Facial (4 mm, 3 mm and 4 mm) and M to D of Lingual (4 mm, 4 mm and 4 mm). Tooth #31 had pain with bite test and pain when occluding. Methylene blue dye and fiber optics showed fracture was through and through and extended below the cementoenamel junction (CEJ).

Diagnostic Tests

Tooth	#29	#30	#31
Percussion	–	–	+
Palpation	–	–	––
Cold	Normal	Normal	–
Mobility	None	None	Class 1
Bite	–	–	+

+: Response to percussion, or bite stick test;
– : No response to percussion, palpation, cold, or on bite stick test

Radiographic Findings

Tooth #31 had a radiolucency that extended from the D cervical area to the apex of the D root. A crack could be seen on the D portion of tooth #31 with the D restorative material fractured. (See Figures 2.1 and 2.2.)

Pretreatment Diagnosis
Pulpal

Pulp Necrosis, tooth #31

Apical

Symptomatic Apical Periodontitis, tooth #31

Treatment Plan
Recommended

Emergency: Extraction, tooth #31
Definitive: Extraction, tooth #31

Alternative

No treatment

Restorative

Implant or Fixed Prosthetics

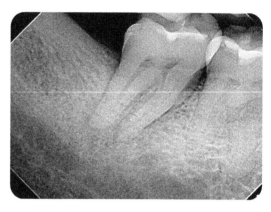

Figure 2.1 The initial radiograph of tooth #31. Notice the shallow restoration and the periapical rarefaction at the root apices.

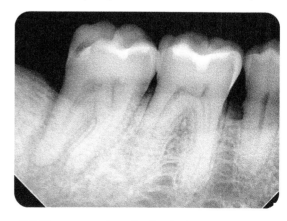

Figure 2.2 The extent of rarefaction in the distal root of tooth #31. Note how the radiolucency moves up to the alveolar crest.

Prognosis

Favorable	Questionable	Unfavorable
		X

Clinical Procedures: Treatment Record

First visit (Day 1): Exam: Pt was referred for an evaluation of tooth #31. Medical history (Hx) and vital signs were taken. Three periapical (PA) radiographs were prescribed in order to evaluate the PA area for possible infection and to determine the extent of the crack. The radiographs showed PA rarefactions (Figures 2.1 and 2.2) at root tips and bone loss in D root area. Clinical tests and exams were performed. Tooth #31 had an M to D crack that was verified with methylene blue (Figure 2.3) and a fiber optic light (Figures 2.4 and 2.5). The tooth could be separated in a buccal–lingual (B–L) manner with light touch. The defect could be seen extending to the pulpal floor. Pt was informed that the prognosis of the tooth was unfavorable and that extraction was needed to alleviate his pain and for healing to occur. The Pt accepted treatment (Tx) of extraction of Tooth #31. The extracted tooth was photographed and confirmed the initial diagnosis of a root fracture and split tooth (Figure 2.6).

Post-Treatment Evaluation

Second visit (1-week follow-up): Pt returned for a post-operative (PO) follow-up. The area around the extraction site of tooth #31 was neither inflamed nor swollen. Gingival tissue had already begun to fill in the socket. The Pt was able to eat and brush his teeth in the lower right quadrant.

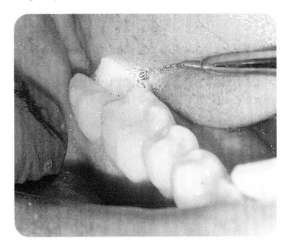

Figure 2.4 Fiber optic light illumination of tooth #31 shows that the crack goes below the CEJ. The light does not pass through from lingual to buccal.

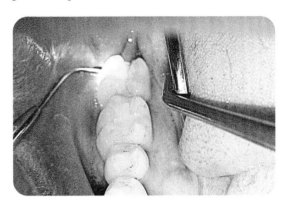

Figure 2.5 Fiber optic light was used on the buccal surface to confirm the crack.

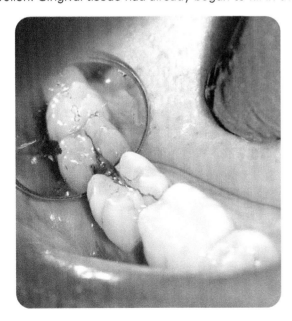

Figure 2.3 Mesial to distal crack of tooth #31, stained with methylene blue to better visualize the extent of the crack.

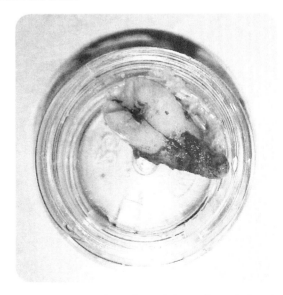

Figure 2.6 Diagnosis of a split tooth is confirmed after the extraction of tooth #31.

Self Study Questions

A. How is a fractured tooth diagnosed?

B. What are the types of cracks one may see in a suspected tooth fracture?

C. What is the prognosis for a cracked tooth?

D. How is a cracked tooth treated?

E. What is the incidence rate of fractures?

Answers to Self-Study Questions

A. There are multiple ways to determine whether or not a tooth is fractured. It is important to start with a good dental history of the tooth. A clinical exam should include a bite stick, ice for vitality testing, and a periodontal probing to check for deep narrow pockets. A radiographic exam is important to check for periapical rarefactions or possibly to reveal a fracture itself if it is large enough. Finally, a stain (methylene blue), or trans-illumination may be used to visualize the fracture. Sometimes the tooth may be mobile or a sinus tract may have developed due to fracture necrosis. If a tooth is non-vital with minimal or no restorations, suspect a crack or fracture (Berman & Kuttler 2010). The older the tooth, the more susceptible it is to fracture (Berman & Kuttler 2010). Cracked teeth are more commonly found in lower molars, followed by maxillary pre-molars (Cameron 1976). Another study found that lower 2nd molars were more likely to have cracks after root canal treatment (Kang, Kim & Kim 2016).

B. According to the American Association of Endodontics (Rivera & Walton 2008), there are five categories of crack:

- Craze lines: Only involving the enamel;
- Split tooth: Complete fracture through the tooth, usually centered mesial to distal;
- Fractured cusp: Usually non-centered and affecting one cusp;
- Cracked tooth: An incomplete fracture that extends from the crown to the subgingival area of the tooth; and
- Vertical Root Fracture (VRF): This may be symptomatic or non- symptomatic. The majority of the VRFs are associated with root-filled teeth. It may be a complete or an incomplete fracture.

C. The prognosis for a cracked tooth is always going to be questionable (Rivera & Walton 2008). The prognosis is always better if the crack does not extend to the pulp chamber floor (Turp & Gobetti 1996; Sim et al. 2016). Vital is better than necrotic (Turp & Gobetti 1996). The quality of the restoration and whether a full coverage crown may cover the crack and other defects are considerations (Rivera & Walton 2008), as is whether an abscess or radiographic rarefaction is present prior to treatment. These two factors would lower the prognosis of the tooth in question (Berman & Kuttler 2010). One study found that cracked teeth had a two-year survival rate of 85.5% (Tan et al. 2006). Another study found that after five years, the survival rate of root-filled cracked teeth was 92%, with the odds of extraction increasing if the cracks were in the root (Sim et al. 2016). Finally, a recent study from Korea showed a 90%, two-year survival rate for a cracked tooth, probing depths greater than 6 mm being a significant factor in the prognosis (Kang et al. 2016).

D. After removal of all caries or previous restorations, the extent of the defect must be determined. If the crack or fracture transverses the pulpal floor or goes too deep subgingivally, then extraction of the tooth must be considered (Sim et al. 2016). If the tooth is vital with no narrow probing defects, abscesses, or periapical rarefactions, then restoring the tooth may be considered, along with endodontic therapy if needed, depending on the health of the pulp (Sim et al. 2016).

If a horizontal fracture occurs due to trauma, the position of the defect and the vitality of the pulp must be evaluated (Andreasen 1970). If the fracture is high enough, the coronal portion may be removed to see if a crown lengthening procedure along with endodontic therapy might salvage the tooth. If the defect is in the apical third, then an RCT to the coronal portion of the root is indicated (Andreasen 1970). If, however, the apical third has a rarefaction, an osteotomy may be performed to remove the infected piece.

Four types of outcome occur with intra-alveolar root fractures: (1) healing with calcified tissue; (2) interposition of connective tissue; (3) interposition of connective tissue and bone; and (4) interposition of granulation tissue without healing (Kim et al. 2016).

E. The incidence rate of VRFs is less than 3% (Zachrisson & Jacobsen 1975), and the rate of crown fractures for all dental trauma is about 2% (Macko *et al.* 1979). Hand instrumentation does not produce dentinal cracks (Yoldas *et al.* 2012). The more tooth structure is removed, the more likely a fracture will occur. It takes about half of the dentin to be removed before cracks begin to appear (Wilcox,

Roskelley & Sutton 1997). A study found that VRFs tend to be more prevalent in maxillary premolars, mandibular molars, women, and individuals over the age of 40. VRFs are more difficult to diagnose because they do not always have deep probing depths (Cohen *et al.* 2006).

References

Andreasen, J. O. (1970) Etiology and pathogenesis of traumatic dental injuries. A clinical study of 1,298 cases. *Scandinavian Journal of Dental Research* **78**, 329–342.

Berman, L. H. & Kuttler, S. (2010) Fracture necrosis: diagnosis, prognosis, assessment, and treatment recommendations. *Journal of Endodontics* **36**, 442–446.

Cameron, C. E. (1976) The cracked tooth syndrome: additional findings. *Journal of the American Dental Association* **93**, 971–975.

Cohen, S., Berman, L. H., Blanco, L. *et al.* (2006) A demographic analysis of vertical root fractures. *Journal of Endodontics* **32**, 1160–1163.

Kang, S. H., Kim, B. S. & Kim, Y. (2016) Cracked teeth: distribution, characteristics, and survival after root canal treatment. *Journal of Endodontics* **42**, 557–562.

Kim, D., Yue, W., Yoon, T. C. *et al.* (2016) Healing of horizontal intra-alveolar root fractures after endodontic treatment with mineral trioxide aggregate. *Journal of Endodontics* **42**, 230–235.

Macko, D. J., Grasso, J. E., Powell, E. A. *et al.* (1979) A study of fractured anterior teeth in a school population. *ASDC Journal of Dentistry for Children* **46**, 130–133.

Rivera, E. & Walton, R. E. (2008) Cracking the cracked tooth code: detection and treatment of various longitudinal tooth fractures. *Endodontics: Colleagues for Excellence Newsletter.* Chicago: American Association of Endodontics.

Sim, I. G., Lim, T. S., Krishnaswamy, G. *et al.* (2016) Decision making for retention of endodontically treated posterior cracked teeth: a 5-year follow-up study. *Journal of Endodontics* **42**, 225–229.

Tan, L., Chen, N. N., Poon, C. Y. *et al.* (2006) Survival of root filled cracked teeth in a tertiary institution. *International Endodontic Journal* **39**, 886–889.

Turp, J. C. & Gobetti J. P. (1996) The cracked tooth syndrome: an elusive diagnosis. *Journal of the American Dental Association* **127**, 1502–1507.

Wilcox, L. R., Roskelley, C. & Sutton, T. (1997) The relationship of root canal enlargement to finger-spreader induced vertical fracture. *Journal of Endodontics* **23**, 533–534.

Yoldas, O., Yilmaz, S., Atakan, G. *et al.* (2012) Dentinal microcrack formation during root canal preparations by different NiTi rotary instruments and the self-adjusting file. *Journal of Endodontics* **38**, 232–235.

Zachrisson, B. U. & Jacobsen, I. (1975) Long term prognosis of 66 permanent anterior teeth with root fracture. *Scandinavian Journal of Dental Research* **83**, 345–354.

3

Diagnostic Case II:
Exploratory Surgery: Repairing Incomplete Fracture

Keivan Zoufan, Takashi Komabayashi, and Qiang Zhu

LEARNING OBJECTIVES
- To understand endodontic diagnoses.
- To understand the etiologic factors of endodontic pathosis.
- To understand the principles and indications of pulpal and apical diagnostic tests.
- To understand the radiographic characteristics of endodontic lesions.
- To understand the concept of exploratory surgery.

	Molars			Premolars		Canine	Incisors				Canine	Premolars		Molars		
							Maxillary arch									
Universal tooth designation system	1	2	3	4	5	6	7	8	9	10	11	12	13	14	15	16
International standards organization designation system	18	17	16	15	14	13	12	11	21	22	23	24	25	26	27	28
Palmer method	8⌋	7⌋	6⌋	5⌋	4⌋	3⌋	2⌋	1⌋	⌊1	⌊2	⌊3	⌊4	⌊5	⌊6	⌊7	⌊8
Palmer method	8⌉	7⌉	6⌉	5⌉	4⌉	3⌉	2⌉	1⌉	⌈1	⌈2	⌈3	⌈4	⌈5	⌈6	⌈7	⌈8
International standards organization designation system	48	47	46	45	44	43	42	41	31	32	33	34	35	36	37	38
Universal tooth designation system	32	31	30	29	28	27	26	25	24	23	22	21	20	19	18	17
							Mandibular arch									
		Right								**Left**						

Clinical Cases in Endodontics, First Edition. Edited by Takashi Komabayashi.
© 2018 John Wiley & Sons, Inc. Published 2018 by John Wiley & Sons, Inc.

Chief Complaint

"I had a root canal re-done on my front tooth, but there's still a bump there. My dentist said maybe it's fractured and sent me to you. By the way, my front teeth are sensitive to cold as well."

Medical History

The patient (Pt) was a 70-year-old female. Vital signs were as follows: Blood pressure (BP) 129/85 mmHg right arm seated (RAS), pulse 63 beats per minute (BPM) and regular, respiratory rate (RR) 16 breaths per minute. No known drug allergies (NKDA). A complete review of systems was conducted. The Pt had controlled seasonal allergies and hypertension and was taking Clarinex® (5 mg daily) for seasonal allergy relief and Zestoretic® (10 mg daily) for high blood pressure treatment.

The Pt was American Society of Anesthesiologists Physical Status Scale (ASA) Class II.

Dental History

The Pt had a history (Hx) of routine dental care. Her oral hygiene was good. Numerous restorations were present. Tooth #7 had been endodontically treated with silver point more than twenty years ago. A sinus tract presented approximately four months ago and a non-surgical retreatment was completed on tooth #7. However, the sinus tract was still present. Pt's general dentist believed that she had a vertical root fracture on tooth #7 and Pt was referred for further evaluation. Two radiographs were provided by her general dentist; one showed tooth #7 had been endodontically treated with silver point and had a normal apex (Figure 3.1).

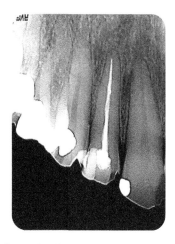

Figure 3.1 Radiograph taken by patient's general dentist 4 months prior to the Pt coming to the office. Tooth #7 had been endodontically treated with silver point.

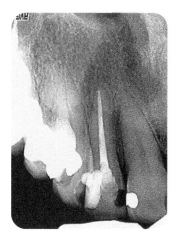

Figure 3.2 Tooth #7 was retreated and the root canal obturation looks adequate.

The second one showed tooth #7 had been retreated and the root canal obturation looked adequate (Figure 3.2).

Clinical Evaluation: (Diagnostic Procedures) Examinations

Pt was alert, normally developed, and was not stressed.

Extra-oral Examination (EOE)

EOE revealed no lymphadenopathy, swelling or sinus tract of the submandibular and neck areas. Soft tissue appeared healthy. Temporomandibular joint (TMJ) was within normal limits (WNL).

Intra-oral Examination (IOE)

A sinus tract was located in the attached gingiva of the labial area between teeth #7 and #8 (Figure 3.3). Periodontal probing depths of teeth #6, #7, #9, and #10 were < 4 mm; however, tooth #8 showed increased pocket depth and bleeding upon probing on middle buccal surface. There had been multiple restorations.

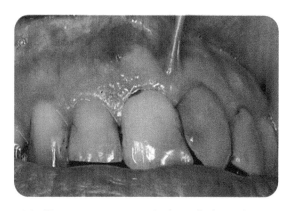

Figure 3.3 Sinus tract was seen in the apical area between teeth #7 and #8.

Tooth #7 was restored with composite; tooth #8 had distal (D) amalgam restoration and discolored BML composite restoration. Discolored ML composite restoration with evidence of recurrent caries was noted on tooth #9. All teeth had normal physiological mobility. Transillumination revealed no cracks or fractures. Placement of Endo Ice® on tooth #8 produced sharp and short sensitivity without lingering pain.

Diagnostic Tests

Tooth	#6	#7	#8	#9
Percussion	–	–	–	–
Palpation	–	–	–	–
Endo Ice®	+	N/A	Sensitivity, no lingering pain	+
EPT	+	N/A	+	+

EPT: Electric pulp test; +: Normal response to Endo Ice® or EPT; –: Normal response to percussion or palpation; N/A: Not applicable

Selective Anesthesia after Diagnostic Tests

Probing on tooth #8 was very painful. Therefore, to assess the exact measurement, local anesthesia using 36 mg lidocaine with 0.018 mg (1:100,000) epinephrine was administered. An 8 mm isolated probing was noted in middle buccal (B) of tooth #8. All other probing depths were <4 mm.

Radiographic Findings

Preoperative radiograph showed teeth #5 and #6 had three surface fillings and normal apical status. Tooth #7 had previous root canal treatment (RCT) and was restored with core build-up. The root filling appeared to be adequate. Normal periradicular structure of teeth #7 and #8 was noted (Figure 3.4). Gutta-percha (GP) tracing

of the sinus tract on B mucosa pointed to D and apical aspect of the root of tooth #8 (Figure 3.5). A GP tracing radiograph showed tooth #8 had mesial (M) and D fillings. A 2 mm × 4 mm lateral lesion extending from 2 mm coronal of the radiographic apex to 6 mm below the alveolar crest was seen on the D surface of tooth #8 (Figure 3.6). The sinus track came from the lesion extending from 2 mm coronal of the radiographic apex to 6 mm below the alveolar crest.

An M restoration of tooth #9 was partially viewed. Also, evidence of recurrent caries was noted (Figure 3.6).

Pretreatment Diagnosis
Pulpal

Reversible Pulpitis, tooth #8

Apical

Normal Apical Tissues, tooth #8

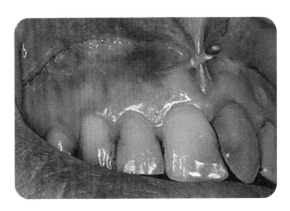

Figure 3.5 Gutta percha traces sinus tract.

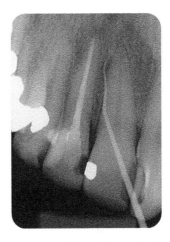

Figure 3.6 Gutta-percha tracing radiograph shows a 2 mm × 4 mm lateral lesion on tooth #8, with the distal surface extending from 2 mm coronal of the radiographic apex to 6 mm below the alveolar crest.

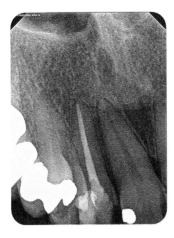

Figure 3.4 Preoperative radiograph shows teeth #7 and #8 have normal apex.

CLINICAL CASES IN ENDODONTICS

Treatment Plan
Recommended
Emergency: No treatment
Definitive: Exploratory surgery of tooth #8. Repairing root crack line (observed in exploratory surgery), and non-surgical root canal treatment (NSRCT) due to the possibility of devitalizing pulp by the crack line repairing procedure.

Alternative
Extraction of tooth #8 or no treatment

Restorative
Core build-up and full coverage restoration

Prognosis

Favorable	Questionable	Unfavorable
	X	

Clinical Procedures: Treatment Record
First visit (Day 1): Exploratory surgery of tooth #8: medical history was reviewed. BP: 129/85 mmHg RAS, pulse 70 BPM. Explained the procedures to the Pt and obtained informed consent. Confirmed with the Pt's physician over phone that for pain control, Tylenol® was more appropriate than ibuprofen because of the beta-blocker drugs that the Pt took for controlling BP. The Pt was concerned about urinary incontinence; assured the Pt that she would be free to go to restroom as needed and that the dental procedure would be as atraumatic as possible. Pt was asked to rinse with 0.12% chlorhexidine. Local anesthesia was administered with two capsules of 2% lidocaine with 1:100,000 epinephrine. A full-thickness sulcular flap from M side of tooth #4 to D side of tooth #10 with a releasing incision M to tooth #4 was elevated. A bony defect in the B side of tooth #8 was noted. The defect perforated the B plate. Also, the interdental alveolar bone was lost on the the B side of tooth #8. Granulation tissue was enucleated and was sent for biopsy. The B surface of tooth #8 was stained with methylene blue and examined at high magnification. A crack line was observed (Figure 3.7). Tooth #7 was fully covered by bone. Because the root apex of tooth #8 was fully surrounded by bone the without the apical lesion seen on PA, and the B lesion did not extend to the root apex, it was decided to repair the crack line. The B crack line was prepared with ultrasonic tips ProUltra® Surgical Endo Tip Size 1 (Dentsply Sirona, Ballaigues, Switzerland)

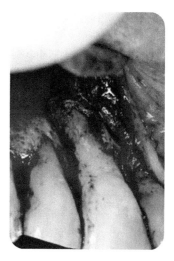
Figure 3.7 A crack line was observed in the root of tooth #8.

under the operative microscope (Global Surgical Corporation, St. Louis, MO, USA) and the prepared groove cavity was filled with Geristore® (DenMat, Lompoc, CA, USA) (Figure 3.8). The flap was well irrigated with 10 ml of 0.9% sodium chloride (NaCl). The wound was closed with 5-0 nylon suture (Nurolon® Suture, Ethicon US LLC, Somerville, NJ, USA). Due to the possibility of devitalizing pulp during the repair procedure, a NSRCT was recommended. The Pt agreed with the recommendation. A rubber dam (RD) and clamp were placed over tooth #8. Restorations were removed with high-speed burs. Access was completed. When the canal was located, the pulp was vital and hyperemic. No evidence of a fracture was noted inside the tooth. A working length (WL) was established and confirmed with a radiograph (Figure 3.9). Instrumentation was performed with Sequence series 0.04 taper rotary files (EndoSequence®, Brasseler USA, Savannah, GA, USA)

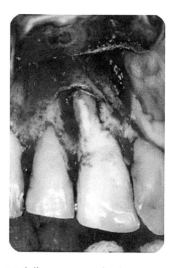
Figure 3.8 The crack line was repaired.

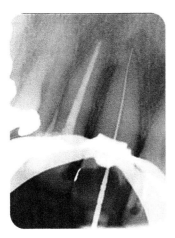

Figure 3.9 Working-length radiograph of tooth #8. Root canal treatment was initiated due to the possibility of devitalizing pulp by the crack-line repairing procedure.

using a crown-down technique. The canal was irrigated with 5 ml of 0.5% sodium hypochlorite (NaOCl) and dried with paper points. A master cone was then placed to length with AH Plus® Root Canal Sealer (Dentsply Sirona, Konstanz, Germany). The canal was obturated by System B™ (Kerr, Orange, CA, USA) and back-filled using Calamus® Dual (Dentsply Sirona, Johnson City, TN, USA). The access cavity was filled with Cavit™ (3M, Two Harbors, MN, USA) and Fuji IX GP® (GC America Inc., Alsip, IL, USA). The RD was removed. Post-operative (PO) vital signs were within normal limit. Post-operative instructions (POI) were given: Peridex™ 0.12% (3M, Two Harbors, MN, USA) rinse two times daily (BID), beginning the second day after surgery for one week. The Pt was instructed to take one tablet Tylenol® 500mg three times daily (TID) as needed (PRN) for pain. Ice pack and gauze were applied. A PO radiograph was made (Figure 3.10).

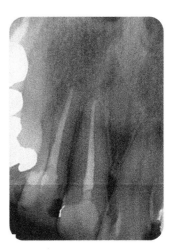

Figure 3.10 Obturation radiograph of tooth #8.

Working length, apical size, and obturation technique

Canal	Working Length	Apical Size	Obturation Materials and Techniques
Single	24.0 mm	45	GP, AH Plus® sealer, Vertical condensation

Second visit (Day 6): Suture removal and biopsy report. RMHX was conducted and vital signs examined. Pt had no swelling and the healing of the surgical wound was uneventful. All sutures were removed. Biopsy reported a cyst lined by hyperplastic unkeratinized stratified squamous epithelium. The wall displayed mild to moderate inflammatory reaction (Figure 3.11). A request was made to Pt's general dentist for a full coverage restoration without a post on tooth #8, as well as caries excavation on tooth #9. A follow-up appointment was scheduled.

Histopathologic Diagnosis

Periapical Cyst (biopsy report)

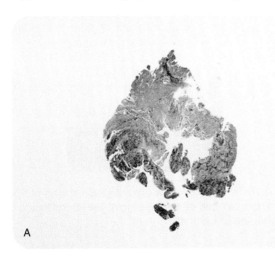

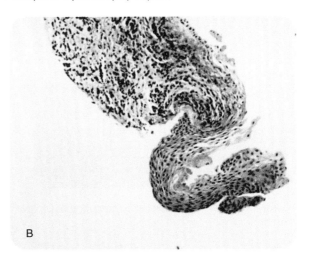

Figure 3.11 Histologic slides of the biopsy tissue revealed a cyst lined by hyperplastic unkeratinized stratified squamous epithelium. The wall contains mild to moderate inflammatory reaction. A: Original magnification ×4; B: Original magnification ×40.

Diagnosis (Post-Treatment)

The cystic lesion was most likely a lateral periodontal cyst considering the cyst was located in the lateral periodontium of tooth #8, and the tooth was vital with normal apex.

Post-Treatment Evaluations

Third visit (1-year follow-up): Pt failed the six-month recall appointment. RMHX. Tooth #8 was asymptomatic and restored with composite core (Filtek™ Supreme Ultra A2B, 3M ESPE, Two Harbors, MN, USA) by her general dentist. The tooth was non-tender to percussion and palpation. A follow-up radiograph was made and it revealed healing of the bony defect (Figure 3.12). The general dentist had performed a RCT on tooth #9 and restored with composite core build-up. Gingiva was normal. Probing depth was <3 mm and mobility was normal. A full-coverage restoration was recommended on teeth #7, #8 and #9. A follow-up appointment was scheduled.

Fourth visit (3-year follow-up): RMHX. Tooth #8 was asymptomatic and non-tender to percussion and palpation. Mobility was normal. Gingiva shape and texture looked normal (Figure 3.13). Probing depth was <3 mm and no bleeding upon probing was noted (Figure 3.14). Apex appeared normal in the periapical (PA) radiograph (Figure 3.15). The Pt was urged to pursue full coverage restoration as soon as possible. Prognosis was favorable.

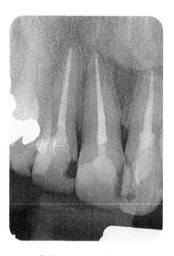

Figure 3.12 One-year follow-up radiograph reveals healing of the lateral lesion on the distal side of tooth #8.

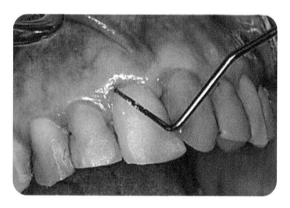

Figure 3.14 Three-year follow-up clinical photograph. No bleeding upon probing.

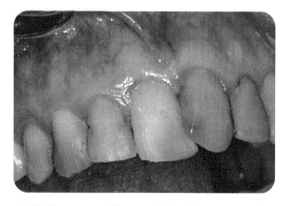

Figure 3.13 Three-year follow-up clinical photograph. Gingiva looks normal.

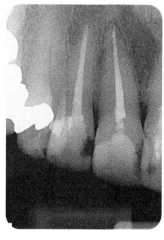

Figure 3.15 Three-year follow-up radiograph shows normal apex of teeth #7 and #8 and healing of the lateral lesion on the distal side of tooth #8.

Self-Study Questions

A. What are the pulpal diagnoses?

B. What are the apical diagnoses?

C. What are the common etiologic factors of endodontic pathosis?

D. What are the common pulp and apical tests?

E. What are the radiographic characteristics of endodontic lesions?

Answers to Self-Study Questions

A. The pulpal diagnoses are (American Association of Endodontists (AAE) Consensus Conference Recommended Diagnostic Terminology 2009; Glickman & Schweitzer 2013):

- **Normal Pulp:** The pulp is vital, has no symptoms and responds normally to pulp testing.
- **Reversible Pulpitis:** The pulp is vital and has short discomfort/pain with a stimulus such as cold or sweet.
- **Symptomatic Irreversible Pulpitis:** The pulp is vital and has spontaneous or lingering or referred pain.
- **Asymptomatic Irreversible Pulpitis:** The pulp is vital and has no symptoms. Pulp exposure may result from trauma, cavity preparation or deep caries.
- **Pulp Necrosis:** The pulp has no response to pulp testing and is asymptomatic.
- **Previously Treated:** The root canals are filled with root canal filling materials.
- **Previously Initiated Therapy:** The tooth has been previously treated by partial endodontic therapy.

B. The apical diagnoses are (AAE Consensus Conference Recommended Diagnostic Terminology 2009; Glickman & Schweitzer 2013):

- **Normal Apical Tissues:** The tooth has no sensitivity to percussion or palpation. Radiograph shows apical normal.
- **Symptomatic Apical Periodontitis:** The tooth has pain to percussion and/or palpation. Radiograph shows apical normal or radiolucency.
- **Asymptomatic Apical Periodontitis:** The tooth has no pain to percussion or palpation. Radiograph shows apical radiolucency due to pulp necrosis.
- **Chronic Apical Abscess:** The tooth has sinus tract. Radiograph shows apical radiolucency due to pulp necrosis.
- **Acute Apical Abscess:** The tooth has spontaneous pain, swelling, pus formation and apical radiolucency due to pulp necrosis.

- **Condensing Osteitis:** Radiograph shows radiopaque lesion.

C. Generally there are etiologic factors in the tooth associated with pulpal and apical pathosis such as caries, crown, restorative filling, cracks, fractures, attrition, abrasion, trauma or developmental abnormalities. If no etiologic factors can be found, it is unlikely the symptoms and/or apical radiolucency are originating from the tooth.

D. The common pulpal tests are electric and thermal pulp testing (Peters, Baumgartner & Lorton 1994; Abbott & Yu 2007). They are used to determine whether the pulp is vital or necrotic. The tooth must be isolated and dried. The electric pulp test probe must contact natural tooth structure. Endo Ice® (1,1,1,2-tetrafluoroethane) is the most-used cold test. The carbon dioxide cone is often used on a tooth with crown or open apex. A heat test is usually reserved for patients complaining of pain with heat. All pulpal tests must have control teeth. Electric and thermal pulp testing are often used at the same time to reduce the possibility of false positive and false negative responses. The common apical tests are percussion and palpation (Abbott & Yu 2007). Either neighboring or contralateral teeth are used as controls. Sinus tract, swelling and periodontal pocket should also be examined for apical diagnosis.

E. Apical lesion due to pulp necrosis has the following characteristics: loss of lamina dura, a hanging drop appearance, and maintenance of the same position on a shifted radiograph. Generally, an etiological factor may be seen on the radiograph. The use of cone beam computed tomography (CBCT) in endodontic treatment should follow the recommendations in the joint position statement of the AAE and the American Academy of Oral and Maxillofacial Radiology (AAOMR) (AAE and AAOMR Joint Position Statement 2015).

References

AAE and AAOMR Joint Position Statement: use of cone beam computed tomography in endodontics 2015 update (2015). *Oral Surgery, Oral Medicine, Oral Pathology and Oral Radiology* **120**, 508–512.

AAE consensus conference recommended diagnostic terminology. (2009) *Journal of Endodontics* **35**, 1634.

Abbott, P.V. & Yu, C. (2007) A clinical classification of the status of the pulp and the root canal system. *Australian Dental Journal* **52** (1 Suppl), S17–S31.

Glickman, G.N. & Schweitzer J.L. (2013) Endodontic diagnosis. *Endodontics: Colleagues for Excellence Newsletter.* American Association of Endodontics, *Chicago: American Association of Endodontics.*

Peters, D.D., Baumgartner, J.C. & Lorton, L. (1994) Adult pulpal diagnosis. I. Evaluation of the positive and negative responses to cold and electrical pulp tests. *Journal of Endodontics* **20**, 506–511.

4

Emergency Case I:
Interprofessional Collaboration between Medical and Dental

Andrew Xu

LEARNING OBJECTIVES

- To understand the role of dental diagnosis in an emergency situation.

- To understand the etiology of endodontic infection and pathogenesis of infection.
- To understand the importance of managing an emergency situation in the endodontics field.

	Molars			Premolars		Canine	Incisors				Canine	Premolars		Molars		
Maxillary arch																
Universal tooth designation system	1	2	3	4	5	6	7	8	9	10	11	12	13	14	15	16
International standards organization designation system	18	17	16	15	14	13	12	11	21	22	23	24	25	26	27	28
Palmer method	8⌋	7⌋	6⌋	5⌋	4⌋	3⌋	2⌋	1⌋	⌊1	⌊2	⌊3	⌊4	⌊5	⌊6	⌊7	⌊8

	Molars			Premolars		Canine	Incisors				Canine	Premolars		Molars		
Palmer method	8⌉	7⌉	6⌉	5⌉	4⌉	3⌉	2⌉	1⌉	⌈1	⌈2	⌈3	⌈4	⌈5	⌈6	⌈7	⌈8
International standards organization designation system	48	47	46	45	44	43	42	41	31	32	33	34	35	36	37	38
Universal tooth designation system	32	31	30	29	28	27	26	25	24	23	22	21	20	19	18	17
Mandibular arch																

Right　　　　　Left

Chief Complaint

"My daughter has a draining fistula on her face and her face has been swollen. What can we do about this?"

Medical History

The patient (Pt) was a 9-year-old Caucasian female. The Pt was healthy with no medical history of note. According to her parents, she was taking Clindamycin. Vital signs were: Blood pressure (BP) 115/68 mmHg, pulse 78 beats per minute (BPM) and regular, respiratory rate (RR) 18 breaths per minute. A temperature of 98.7° F was taken sublingually. A complete review of systems was conducted. No significant findings were noted, and there were no contraindications to dental treatment.

The Pt was classified as American Society of Anesthesiologist Physical Status Scale (ASA) Class I.

Dental History

The Pt's mother stated that the Pt had a filling completed on tooth #19 a year ago. The Pt developed a toothache in the area three months ago and went to the general dentist to seek treatment (Tx). The general dentist stated that the tooth #19 did not require any Tx and that the pain was coming from tooth #18 due to eruption. No Tx was performed at the time. A few weeks later, the Pt developed left facial swelling and an extra-oral sinus tract (Figures 4.1 and 4.2). The Pt went to seek treatment at an otolaryngologist (ENT) office. The ENT drained the sinus tract (Figure 4.3), prescribed antibiotics and referred the Pt to the endodontic clinic. The Pt had spontaneous moderate pain while at the endodontic clinic.

Figure 4.1 Preoperative photograph, before drainage procedure by an otolaryngologist.

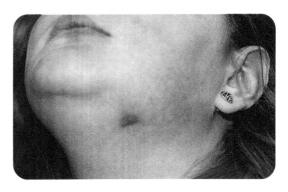

Figure 4.2 Preoperative photograph during the emergency appointment.

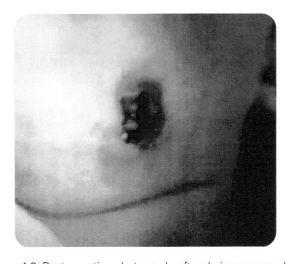

Figure 4.3 Postoperative photograph, after drainage procedure on the sinus tract by an otolaryngologist.

Clinical Evaluation (Diagnostic Procedures)
Examinations
Extra-oral Examination (EOE)

Examination showed facial swelling associated with the left mandible, extending to the inferior border of the mandible. Slight facial asymmetry was noted, with erythematous appearance over the cheek in the affected area. The left submandibular gland region and lymph nodes were palpable, moveable and tender. The temporomandibular joint (TMJ) demonstrated no discomfort to opening or closing, and no popping or clicking or deviation to either side upon opening. An extra-oral sinus tract was noted, and scar tissue had formed around the facial sinus track.

Intra-oral Examination (IOE)

Examination showed a fluctuant swelling in the area of the apices of the roots of tooth #19 with distension of the vestibular tissues.

Diagnostic Tests

Tooth	#18	#19	#20
Percussion	–	+	N/A
Palpation	–	+	–
Cold	+	–	N/A
EPT	+	–	N/A

EPT: Electric pulp test; + : Severe response to percussion and palpation, normal response to cold and EPT; – : No response to percussion, palpation, cold, or EPT; N/A: Not applicable

Radiographic Findings

An initial periapical radiograph of tooth #19 was taken (Figure 4.4) which yielded a partial view of tooth #18. Tooth #19 had a deep occlusal restoration close to the mesial (M) pulp horn. The pretreatment radiograph demonstrated a small, well-defined periapical radiolucency (PARL) involving the distal (D) root apex. There was a widened periodontal ligament (PDL) around M root. Pt also had a radix entomolaris root on the distal (D) side of the tooth.

Pretreatment Diagnosis
Pulpal

Pulp Necrosis, tooth #19

Apical

Acute Apical Abscess, tooth #19

Treatment Plan
Recommended

Emergency: Pulp Debridement and placement of calcium hydroxide (Ca(OH)₂)

Definitive: Non-surgical Root Canal Therapy (NSRCT)

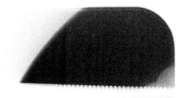
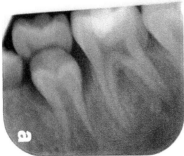

Figure 4.4 Preoperative radiograph.

Alternative

Extraction or no treatment

Restorative

Core build-up and stainless steel crown until permanent crown can be placed

Prognosis

Favorable	Questionable	Unfavorable
X		

Clinical Procedures: Treatment Record

First visit (Day 1): Pt's medical history was reviewed (RMHX) and informed consent was obtained. The endodontic evaluation and treatment plan were discussed with the Pt's parents; alternative Txs were discussed. Local anesthesia was obtained by inferior alveolar nerve block (IANB) and long buccal infiltration using 72 mg of 2% Xylocaine with 1:100,000 (0.036 mg) epinephrine (epi). The tooth was isolated with rubber dam (RD) placement and then access was made using a #330 carbide bur using a high-speed hand-piece under copious water. A non-vital pulp was noted. An Endo-Z® bur (Dentsply Sirona, Ballaigues, Switzerland) was used to de-roof the pulp chamber. Copious irrigation was conducted using sodium hypochlorite (NaOCl). M buccal (B), M lingual (L), DB, DL were found with the use of a dental operating microscope (Global Surgical Corporation, St. Louis, MO, USA). No evidence was observed of any fractures inside the tooth. The canals were negotiated with a size #10 hand stainless steel Lexicon® K-file (Dentsply Sirona, Johnson City, TN, USA) and a chelating agent (RC-Prep®; Premier Dental Products, Morristown, PA, USA). Working length (WL) was obtained using an electronic apex locator (Root ZX®II, J. Morita, Kyoto, Japan) and recorded. MB canal length of 19 mm was obtained using MB cusp, ML canal length of 18.5 mm was obtained using ML cusp, DB canal length of 20 mm was obtained using DB cusp, and DL canal length of 18 mm was obtained using DL cusp. The canals were cleaned and shaped with NiTi rotary instrument (EndoSequence®; Brasseler USA, Savannah, GA, USA) to size #35, .04 taper on the MB and ML canals. DB and DL were prepared to size #40, .04 taper. Canals were dried with paper points. Ca(OH)₂ (Ultracal® XS; Ultradent, South Jordan, UT, USA) was applied as an inter-appointment medicament. Cavit™ (3M, Two Harbors, MN, USA) was used for a temporary seal to the coronal access. The occlusion was examined and adjusted (Figure 4.5). Postoperative instruction (POI) was given. Pt was scheduled for next appointment.

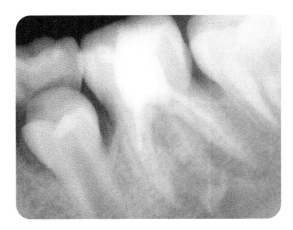

Figure 4.5 Postoperative radiograph after the initial emergency treatment (pulp debridement and placement of calcium hydroxide).

Second visit (Day 13): RMHX. BP 109/67 mmHg, pulse 70 BPM and regular. The Pt presented as asymptomatic, with no signs of extra-oral swelling. A preoperative radiograph was taken (Figure 4.6). Local anesthesia was achieved with 72 mg. of 2% Xylocaine with 1:100,000 (0.036mg) epinephrine by IANB and B infiltration to tooth #19. A single tooth isolation was exercised with RD, temporary restorations were removed, and canals and chamber were irrigated with copious 2.5% NaOCl. The canals were dried with paper points. WL was re-established with an electronic apex locator. All canals were re-instrumented with NiTi rotary instruments, and master cones were fitted and verified with radiograph. The canals were obturated by vertical warm method by using gutta-percha (GP) and Roth's 801 (Grossman type) sealer (Figures 4.7 and 4.8). Amalgam was used as a final restoration. Occlusion was examined and the final radiograph was taken. POI was given and Pt was

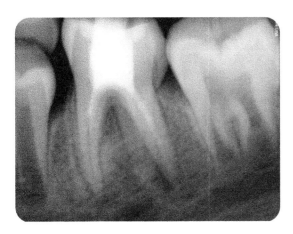

Figure 4.6 Preoperative radiograph for the second visit after 13 days of calcium hydroxide treatment. Patient was asymptomatic at this appointment.

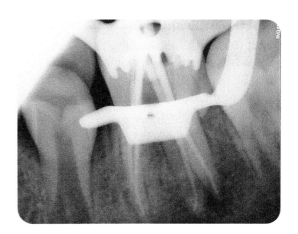

Figure 4.7 Master cone radiograph with gutta percha.

advised to take children's ibuprofen as needed for pain. The Pt was referred back to her dentist for any further Tx. Sealer extruded beyond the apex of the radix entomolaris root on radiograph needed to be monitored during follow-up.

Working length, apical size, and obturation technique

Canal	Working Length	Apical Size	Obturation Materials and Techniques
MB	19.0 mm	35	GP, Roth's 801 sealer, Vertical warm compaction
ML	18.5 mm	35	GP, Roth's 801 sealer, Vertical warm compaction
DB	20.0 mm	40	GP, Roth's 801 sealer, Vertical warm compaction
DL	18.0 mm	40	GP, Roth's 801 sealer, Vertical warm compaction

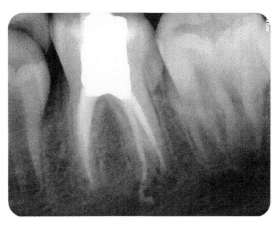

Figure 4.8 Final radiograph with gutta percha and amalgam core build-up.

Post-Treatment Evaluation

Third visit (6-month follow-up): Pt came in for a six-month recall examination. She remained asymptomatic, EOE and IOE revealed no swelling, and tissue appeared healthy. Pt's scar tissue development on her left side of neck area was still present (Figure 4.9). A periapical (PA) radiograph was taken (Figure 4.10). PDL and bone pattern were within normal limit (WNL). Pt's parent had taken the Pt to see a dermatologist for the evaluation for the scar tissue in the previously facial sinus track region. Dermatologist's report stated that Pt's parent declined any Tx for the scar tissue.

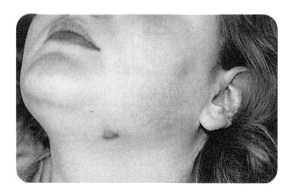

Figure 4.9 Six-month recall photograph.

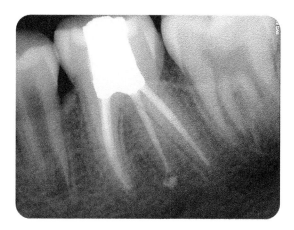

Figure 4.10 Six-month recall radiograph.

Self-Study Questions

A. Does the size of radiolucency in the periapical regions correlate to the severity of an infection?

B. Can an extra-oral sinus tract heal on its own after surgical intervention to drain/clean it?

C. Can a tooth with an acute apical abscess test positive with a cold test?

D. What is the etiology of the infection for the case in this chapter?

E. What could be done to prevent the misdiagnosis that was made by the patient's general dentist in this chapter?

Answers to Self-Study Questions

A. The size of radiolucency in the periapical regions has no correlation to the severity of an infection. A clinician should not rely solely on a radiograph to diagnose a case. Several factors, such as the pathway of bone resorption and the amount of the bone resorption and locations of the roots, all can contribute the appearance of radiolucency in a conventional digital radiograph (Bender 1997).

B. If the tooth is the source of infection that caused the extra-oral sinus tract, the sinus tract or infection will not heal even after surgical intervention to curettage the sinus tract (Goldberg & Topazian 1981). The infected tooth must be treated (Kakehashi, Stanley & Fitzgerald 1965).

C. Generally speaking, a tooth that develops a sinus tract should test negative with a cold test. However, one needs to be aware that a patient can still give a false positive response with a cold test due to residual pulp tissue remaining (Yamasaki *et al.* 1994). When a patient is in moderate to severe pain, pulpal thermal tests may not be a reliable source (Chambers 1982).

D. The etiology of the infection in the illustrated case in this chapter was bacterial (Kakehashi *et al.* 1965). The most likely passage was the junction between the composite and enamel. The preparation site might also have been contaminated during restoration procedures. Streptococcus bacteria are 0.5–2.0 micrometer in diameter. An average middle dentinal tubule diameter size is 1.2 micrometer and 2.5 micrometer near the pulp chamber. If there is bacterial contamination in the cavity preparation site, bacteria can penetrate into the pulp through dentinal tubules (Michelich, Schuster & Pashley 1980).

E. Radiographs alone should not be used for endodontic diagnosis (Bender & Seltzer 1961; Bender 1997). The clinician should listen carefully to the patient's chief complaint, and carry out thorough intra- and extra-oral exams. The new technology of cone beam-computed tomography (CBCT) can also be a very helpful tool to help diagnose difficult cases (Lascala, Panella & Marques 2004).

References

Bender, I. B. (1997) Factors influencing the radiographic appearance of bony lesions. *Journal of Endodontics* **23**, 5–14.

Bender, I. B., & Seltzer, S. (1961) Roentgenographic and direct observation of experimental lesions in bone: I. *The Journal of the American Dental Association* **62**, 152–160.

Chambers, I. G. (1982) The role and methods of pulp testing in oral diagnosis: a review. *International Endodontic Journal* **15**, 1–15.

Goldberg, M. H. & Topazian, R. G. (eds.) (1981) *Odontogenic Infections and Deep Fascial Space Infections of Dental Origin: Management of Infections of the Oral and Maxillofacial Regions*, p. 173. Philadelphia: W.B. Saunders.

Kakehashi, S., Stanley, H. R. & Fitzgerald R. J. (1965) The effects of surgical exposures of dental pulps in germ-free and conventional laboratory rats. *Oral Surgery, Oral Medicine, Oral Pathology* **20**, 340–349.

Lascala, C. A., Panella, J. & Marques, M. M. (2004) Analysis of the accuracy of linear measurements obtained by cone beam-computed tomography (CBCT-NewTom). *Dentomaxillofacial Radiology* **33**, 291–294.

Michelich, V. J., Schuster, G. S. & Pashley, D. H. (1980) Bacterial penetration of human dentin *in vitro*. *Journal of Dental Research* **59**, 1398–1403.

Yamasaki, M., Kumazawa, M., Kohsaka, T. *et al.* (1994) Pulpal and periapical tissue reactions after experimental pulpal exposure in rats. *Journal of Endodontics* **20**, 13–17.

5

Emergency Case II:
Pulpal Debridement, Incision and Drainage (Intra-oral)

Victoria E. Tountas

LEARNING OBJECTIVES
- To be able to properly diagnose a necrotic pulp case based on clinical and radiographic criteria.
- To understand the etiology of infection and pain in a necrotic pulp case.
- To effectively address and provide relief in a necrotic case, on an emergency basis.

	Molars			Premolars		Canine	Incisors				Canine	Premolars		Molars		
							Maxillary arch									
Universal tooth designation system	1	2	3	4	5	6	7	8	9	10	11	12	13	14	15	16
International standards organization designation system	18	17	16	15	14	13	12	11	21	22	23	24	25	26	27	28
Palmer method	8⏌	7⏌	6⏌	5⏌	4⏌	3⏌	2⏌	1⏌	⏌1	⏌2	⏌3	⏌4	⏌5	⏌6	⏌7	⏌8
Palmer method	8⏋	7⏋	6⏋	5⏋	4⏋	3⏋	2⏋	1⏋	⏋1	⏋2	⏋3	⏋4	⏋5	⏋6	⏋7	⏋8
International standards organization designation system	48	47	46	45	44	43	42	41	31	32	33	34	35	36	37	38
Universal tooth designation system	32	31	30	29	28	27	26	25	24	23	22	21	20	19	18	17
							Mandibular arch									
		Right										**Left**				

Clinical Cases in Endodontics, First Edition. Edited by Takashi Komabayashi.
© 2018 John Wiley & Sons, Inc. Published 2018 by John Wiley & Sons, Inc.

Chief Complaint

"My tooth started hurting really bad yesterday. Today I woke up swollen. I can't even touch the tooth with my tongue; the pain is excruciating."

Medical History

The patient (Pt) was a 42-year-old male who had hypertension and was at the time on Hydrochlorothiazide/ Valsartan 160 mg/12 mg per os per day. No known drug allergies (NKDA) were reported. Previous physical examination had been within the preceding six months.

The Pt was American Society of Anesthesiologists Physical Status Scale (ASA) Class II.

Dental History

The Pt reported that tooth #19 had received a porcelain-fused-to-metal (PFM) crown approximately two years previously. Pt started experiencing pain the previous day, and the pain rapidly intensified overnight. Pt noted extra-oral swelling on his lower left (LL) quadrant on the morning of his visit to this office (Figure 5.1). The pain was severe, constant and throbbing in nature; spontaneous and aggravated by mastication and pressure; and was intensified with supination. The pain localized to tooth #19 (The Pt pointed to offending tooth). The Pt had also been experiencing referred pain to his left ear. The Pt had not been able to get relief after four tablets of Ibuprofen 200 mg.

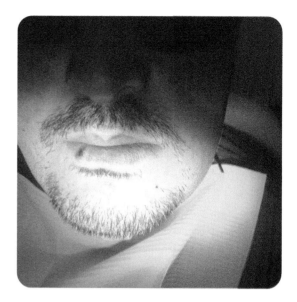

Figure 5.2 Extra-oral swelling on LL with asymmetry.

Clinical Evaluation
Examinations
Extra-oral Examination (EOE)

There was facial swelling in the LL quadrant (Figure 5.2); The temporomandibular joint (TMJ) showed no popping, clicking or deviation on opening; lymph nodes were not swollen.

Intra-oral Examination (IOE)

Soft tissue was erythematous (Figure 5.3); with swelling. There was no sinus tract and oral hygiene was fair. The Pt had a PFM crown on tooth #19.

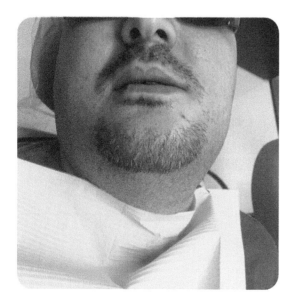

Figure 5.1 Pt presents with extra-oral swelling on LL quadrant and facial asymmetry.

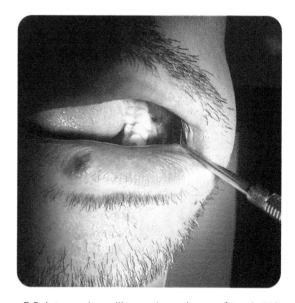

Figure 5.3 Intra-oral swelling on buccal area of tooth #19. Gingival tissues are erythematous.

Diagnostic Tests

Tooth	#19	#18
Percussion	+++	–
Palpation	+++	+
Cold	–	+
Heat	Not performed	Not performed
Mobility	Grade 1	0
Bite Stick	+++	+
Discoloration	None	None
Periodontal Examination		
Probing Depth	4 mm	3 mm
Recession	0	0
Furcation	0	0
Bleed Probing	+++	++

+++: Significant response to percussion, palpation and bite stick and significant probe bleeding.

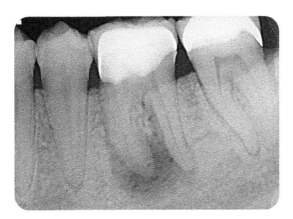

Figure 5.4 Preoperative radiograph of tooth #19. Tooth #19 presents with PFM crown, large PAR on M root and smaller PAR on D root. MB and ML canals appear calcified.

Radiographic Findings

Tooth #19 presented with PFM crown (Figure 5.4). Teeth #18 (partially visible), #20 and #21 (partially visible) were also present. Large periapical radiolucency (PAR) noted on mesial (M) root. Radiolucency extended to mid-root level. M root appeared severely calcified. Distal (D) root presented with PAR. The pulpal chamber appeared calcified. Crestal bone appeared intact. Tooth #18 also presented with PFM crown. Mesial root of tooth #18 presented with periodontal ligament space (PDL) widening.

Pretreatment Diagnosis
Pulpal

Pulp Necrosis, tooth #19

Apical

Acute Apical Abscess, tooth #19

Treatment Plan
Recommended

Emergency: Emergency palliative debridement (open and medicate), and Incision and Drainage (I&D)
Definitive: Non-surgical root canal treatment (NSRCT)

Alternative

Extraction, no treatment

Restorative

Build-up

Prognosis

Favorable	Questionable	Unfavorable
X		

Clinical Procedures: Treatment Record

First visit (Day 1): Reviewed medical history (RMHX). Blood pressure (BP) was 131/98 mmHg, pulse 101 beats per minute (BPM) and regular. Treatment (Tx) plan was reviewed and informed consent was obtained. Operations: Emergency palliative debridement (open and medicate). Anesthesia and rubber dam isolation (RDI): topical anesthesia was obtained with benzocaine (20%) placed on buccal gingiva of tooth #19; lidocaine (lido) 2% with 1:100,000 epinephrine (epi) was given via inferior alveolar nerve block (IANB) (one carpule); articaine 4% with 1:100,000 epi was given via local infiltration on B gingiva, at the height of tooth #19 apices (one carpule). 10 minutes was allowed for anesthetic to take effect.

Pt reported numbness on left side of tongue and lower lip. Anesthesia was verified with application of explorer to B and L gingiva of tooth #19. Pt reported no sensation.

A medium-sized bite block was placed on Pt's right side. A latex RDI was placed. OraSeal® (Ultradent Products, Inc., South Jordan, UT, USA) used on buccal (B) and lingual (L) surfaces to enhance isolation. A #14 RD clamp was used (Hu-Friedy, Chicago, IL, USA). Access was created through PFM crown with extra coarse diamond and Transmetal burs (Dentsply Sirona, Ballaigues, Switzerland) and refined with Endo-Z® bur (Dentsply Sirona, Ballaigues, Switzerland). A counterbalance was used to minimize discomfort to the Pt's TMJ. Magnification and enhanced lighting were used throughout the procedure.

Heavy purulence was noted upon accessing pulpal chamber (Figure 5.5). Copious amounts of sodium hypochlorite (NaOCl) were used as an irrigant to facilitate drainage.

In cleaning and shaping, three separate canals were identified using endodontic explorer: mesiobuccal (MB), mesiolingual (ML) and D.

Initial scouting of canals was performed with stainless steel (SS) size #8 K-files. An electronic apex locator was used to determine canal lengths. All canals were patent. Canals were cleaned and shaped (C&S) using a combination of rotary and hand files. The cleaning and shaping procedure was initiated by enlarging the canal orifices with nickel–titanium (NiTi) orifice shaper rotary files. Copious amounts of NaOCl were used as irrigant throughout the procedure.

All canals exhibited slight curvature, and mesial canals were calcified. Instrumentation was performed using a hybrid technique. Electropolished NiTi rotary files were used, in conjunction with SS hand files (size #10), to verify patency. Following initial shaping up to size #20, .04 taper, purulence stopped and hemorrhage was noted through all canals (Figure 5.6).

MB and ML canals C&S to size #30, .04 taper at 21.0 mm. D canal was C & S to size #40, .04 taper at 20.5 mm.

Calcium hydroxide (Ca(OH)$_2$) placement, temporary restoration and I&D: All canals were dried with paper points. Dry conditions were achieved with minimal hemorrhage still present in D canal. Ca(OH)$_2$ was placed using an engine-driven Lentulo® Spiral Filler (Dentsply Sirona, Ballaigues, Switzerland). Proper distribution of

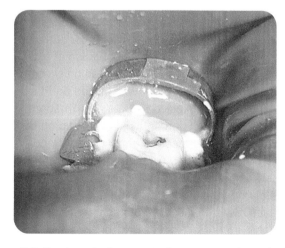

Figure 5.5 Purulent discharge noted upon accessing pulpal chamber. RDI in place with tooth #14. RD clamp and OraSeal® on B and L surfaces.

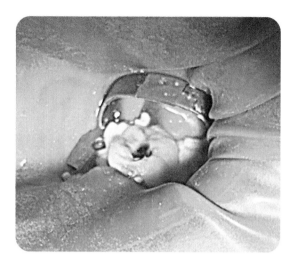

Figure 5.6 Hemorrhage noted after initial C&S, under RDI.

Ca(OH)$_2$ was verified by radiograph (Figure 5.7). Extrusion of Ca(OH)$_2$ was noted radiographically on M root.

The tooth was temporized with cotton and Cavit™ (3M, Two Harbors, MN, USA). The intra-oral swelling was incised with 15C scalpel at the most fluctuant point. Purulent and hemorrhagic discharge were noted (Figure 5.8). Digital pressure was applied to surrounding structures to facilitate drainage.

Pt was prescribed Ibuprofen 800mg / 6 hours, Amoxicillin 500 mg q8h (t.i.d.) and Chlorhexidine 0.12% (rinse). Pt was instructed to return in one week for completion of treatment, but to contact us if symptoms persisted or worsened.

Second visit (Day 7): Operations: NS-RCT: Pt presented asymptomatic, without intra-oral or extra-oral swelling.

Anesthesia and RDI: RMHX. BP was 123/87 mmHg, pulse 86 BPM and regular. Tx plan was reviewed and informed consent was obtained.

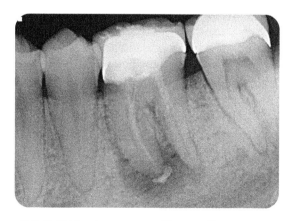

Figure 5.7 Ca(OH)$_2$ placement verification. Extrusion noted on M root. D canal appears filled to mid-root level.

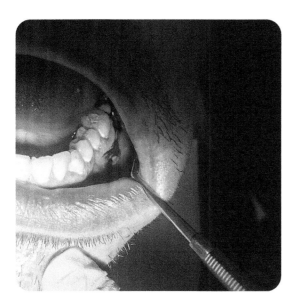

Figure 5.8 I&D performed on buccal gingiva. Hemorrhage and purulent discharge noted.

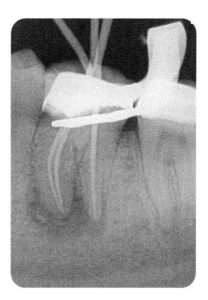

Figure 5.9 Master cone fit radiograph of tooth #19.

Topical anesthesia was applied (Benzocaine 20%) and placed on buccal gingiva of tooth #19. Lido 2% with 1:100K epi was given via IANB (1 carpule). Articaine 4% with 1:100K epi was given via local infiltration on B gingiva, at the height of tooth #19 apices (1 carpule). 10 minutes was allowed for anesthetic to take effect.

Pt reported numbness on left side of tongue and lower lip. Anesthesia was verified with application of explorer to B and L gingiva of tooth #19; Pt reported no sensation.

A medium size bite block was placed on Pt's right side and a latex RDI placed. OraSeal® was used on B and L surfaces; to enhance isolation, a #14 RD clamp was used (Hu-Friedy, Chicago, IL, USA). Cavit™ was removed with diamond bur and the cotton pellet was retrieved with an explorer. A counterbalance was used to minimize discomfort to the Pt's TMJ. Magnification and enhanced lighting were used throughout the procedure.

No purulence was noted. Copious amounts of NaOCl were used as irrigant to remove remaining Ca(OH)$_2$. MB and ML canals were further C&S to size #35, .04 taper at 21.0 mm. EDTA was used as final irrigating solution, to allow for smear layer removal.

Obturation and Temporary Restoration: All canals were dried with paper points. Dry conditions were achieved, without drainage noted. Gutta-percha (GP) points were selected based on the size of the final

apical preparation and a master cone radiograph was obtained (Figure 5.9).

Canals were filled with warm vertical compaction (WVC), using AH26® Root Canal Sealer (Dentsply Sirona, Konstanz, Germany). Canal orifices were sealed with flowable composite to prevent contamination, and the tooth was temporized with cotton and Cavit™ (Figure 5.10). Small sealer extrusion (puff) was noted on the M root. Tooth #19 treatment was completed uneventfully.

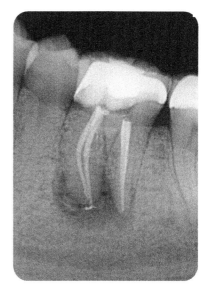

Figure 5.10 Postoperative radiograph of tooth #19, with sealer puff on M root.

Working length, apical size, and obturation technique

Canal	Working Length	Apical Size, Taper	Obturation Materials and Techniques
MB	21.0 mm	35, .04	GP and AH26® sealer, WVC
ML	21.0 mm	35, .04	GP and AH26® sealer, WVC
DB	20.5 mm	40, .04	GP and AH26® sealer, WVC

The Pt was given the option to take a break during the procedure. He was told to return to general dentist for permanent restoration of tooth #19. The patient was informed that tooth might need extraction if not permanently restored upon completion of endodontic Tx.

Post-Treatment Evaluations

None available. Pt was a sailor and left the country the day after Tx was completed.

Self-study Questions

A. What information from the clinical and radiographic examination will lead to the diagnosis of pulp necrosis? What clinical presentations can appear?

B. Which microorganisms have been found to cause infection in necrotic cases?

C. What is the first line of defense to treating an emergency stemming from a necrotic pulp?

D. What are the basic objectives and principles in cleaning and shaping a canal?

E. Should a tooth be left open?

Answers to Self-Study Questions

A. A tooth with a necrotic pulp can manifest as an emergency in any of the following ways:
1. Acute Apical Periodontitis (AAP) without swelling
2. Acute Apical Abscess (AAA) with fluctuant swelling (draining may or may not be present)
3. Diffuse Facial Swelling with or without drainage through canal system (Wolcott, Rossman & Hasselgeren 2011).

Upon interviewing a patient experiencing intense symptoms, our priority should be to determine the chief complaint (CC). In this case, the CC was pain. Secondly, the history and nature of said pain needs to be evaluated. A tooth with pulp necrosis will not respond to cold testing, except in cases of liquefaction necrosis or necrobiosis (partial necrosis) in multi-rooted teeth. Percussion will be positive, signifying the spread of inflammation to the periradicular tissues. Palpation will also likely be positive, as will examination with a bite stick.

The nature of pain associated with a necrotic tooth presenting as an emergency will involve constant moderate to severe pain. It could be spontaneously produced, or triggered by stimulation, such as percussion or mastication. Supination could aggravate symptomatology, while the pain could have throbbing characteristics.

The pain could be localized in the specific tooth, or be diffuse, involving an entire quadrant, and even refer to other anatomical areas (ear, throat, eye) (Glick 1962).

The radiographic findings can present a wide range, depending on the duration of necrosis and stage of inflammation. A necrotic tooth can present with a normal periapical area, a widened or obscure PDL or a clear radiolucent area. It can also manifest with condensing osteitis or resorption of the root structure.

The extra-oral exam can reveal facial swelling with asymmetry and swollen nodes in the affected area. During the intra-oral exam, the clinical crown can present with an existing restoration, caries, traumatic pulpal exposure or fracture. Soft tissues can present with or without swelling. The presence of a sinus tract depends on the duration and intensity of the disease.

B. A tooth presenting with pulp necrosis that has never been accessed before will fall under the category of primary intraradicular infection. In primary infections, the necrotic pulp tissue becomes colonized by a mix of 10–30 taxa of microorganisms (Siqueira & Rocas 2005).

It has been noted that the larger the size of periapical destruction, the greater the bacterial diversity. The bacteria dominating the infected canals are primarily Gram-negative anaerobes, particularly rods, such as *Tannerella*, *Porphyromonas*, *Prevotella*, *Fusobacterium* and *Treponema* (spirochetes). Some Gram-positive anaerobes, such as certain cocci (*Streptococcus*, *Peptostreptococcus*, *Enterococcus*) and rods (*Actinomyces*, *Propionibacterium*, *Lactobacillus*) can also be found in primary infections, as can facultative or microaerophilic streptococci. Certain viruses (HIV, HSV) and fungi (*Candida*) have also been found in primary endodontic infections (Sedgley 2011).

Some Gram-negative anaerobic species have been linked to symptomatic cases; however, data suggests that these species can also be found in asymptomatic cases.

C. It has been established that acute apical periodontitis (AAP) and acute apical abscesses (AAA) are caused by microorganisms and their byproducts egressing the infected root canal system, and communicating with the periodontal tissues. The first line of defense in treating cases presenting with AAP is the removal of these microbes, as well as their byproducts, from the canal system. By effectively debriding the canal system, the stimuli causing apical periodontitis are removed and the inflammatory process can begin to shut down (Peters & Peters 2011).

Microbial elimination in cases with necrotic pulp can be achieved through mechanical instrumentation (debridement), irrigation with disinfecting solutions (NaOCl, CHX, EDTA) and placement of intracanal medications (Ca(OH)$_2$) (Law & Messer 2004; Sathorn, Parashos & Messer 2007). Canal debridement is considered the first line of defense in these cases, as instrumentation alone, even without disinfectants, reduces the existing flora by up to 90% (Dalton *et al.* 1980). According to recent studies, debridement results in a statistically significant reduction in post-operative pain, when compared to the sole prescription of medication without clinical intervention.

While most microbes in an intraradicular infection can be found in a fluid phase, some microorganisms form biofilms that penetrate the dentinal tubules and extend to varying depths into dentin. Files that engage the dentinal walls literally "scrape" and disrupt the microbial biofilm, and remove necrotic pulp tissue, thus eliminating the cause of disease (Love, McMillan & Jenkinson 1997).

The material of the instruments used to clean and shape the canal system has not been found to affect total microbial reduction. Rather, the final shape of the canal is important with regards to the number of remaining bacteria (Card *et al.* 2002).

D. The basic objectives in cleaning and shaping are:
- Removal of infected soft and hard tissue
- Granting apical access to medicaments and disinfecting solutions
- Creation of space for obturation
- Retention of integrity of radicular structure, preventing vertical fractures (Peters & Peters 2011)

A multitude of files can be used for the debridement of the canal system. These include, but are not limited to: K-files, reamers, Hedstrom files, broaches, C+ files, Gates Glidden drills, Peeso reamers, NiTi, stainless steel (SS) files, M wire files, controlled memory files. Traditionally, hand files have been used to establish a glide path at the beginning of treatment. Rotaries can be used on a

canal-specific basis, utilizing their strengths. Larger taper rotaries are typically used for orifice shaping, whereas less tapered files offer more flexibility, respect the anatomy of the canals and deliver safe apical enlargement. Rotary files can be used in a continuous rotary or a reciprocating mode.

Although the removal of all infected dentin is not currently feasible, as all root canal surfaces cannot be mechanically prepared, there are multiple techniques to help overcome this limitation.

Most commonly preferred techniques involve some method of coronal enlargement, followed by different middle and apical third preparation sequences and sizes/ tapers. Special attention needs to be paid to the apical area as the larger the apex, the more volume of disinfectant delivered (Card *et al.* 2002; Souza 2006).

Each clinician needs to address individually the specific needs of each canal system, trying to respect and maintain the original anatomy, remaining mindful of the vast anatomic variations, not only between different individuals, but among different teeth and even different roots and canals.

E. Historically, leaving a tooth open between visits, for the purpose of drainage, was common practice (Torabinejad *et al.* 1988). Based on current studies, this practice is no longer recommended, as it can lead to more complications and inferior success rates in the long-term prognosis of treatment (Simon, Chimenti & Mintz 1982). If a tooth is left open, foreign objects can gain entry to the periapical tissues, and opportunistic bacteria, hereto without access to the canal system, can colonize the radicular dentin. This can lead to a secondary intraradicular infection and reduce chances of successful elimination of microbial flora.

References

Card, S.J., Sigurdsson, A., Orstavik, D. *et al.* (2002) The effectiveness of increased apical enlargement in reducing intracanal bacteria. *Journal of Endodontics* **28**, 779–783.

Dalton, B.C., Orstavik, D., Phillips, C. *et al.* (1980) Bacterial reduction with nickel-titanium rotary instrumentation. *Journal of Endodontics* **24**, 763–767.

Glick, D.H. (1962) Locating referred pulpal pains. *Oral Surgery, Oral Medicine, Oral Pathology* **15**, 613–623.

Law, A. & Messer, H. (2004) An evidence-based analysis of the antibacterial effectiveness of intracanal medicaments. *Journal of Endodontics* **30**, 689–694.

Love, R.M., McMillan, M.D. & Jenkinson, H. F. (1997) Invasion of dentinal tubules by oral streptococci is associated with collagen recognition mediated by the antigen I/II family of polypeptides. *Infection and Immunity* **65**, 5157–5164.

Peters, O.A. & Peters, C.I. (2011) Cleaning and shaping of the root canal system. *Cohen's Pathways of the Pulp* (eds. K. Hargreaves & S. Cohen), 10th edn, pp. 283–248. St. Louis, MO: Elsevier.

Sathorn, C., Parashos, P. & Messer, H. (2007) Antibacterial efficacy of calcium hydroxide intracanal dressing: a systematic review and meta-analysis. *International Endodontic Journal* **40**, 2–10.

Sedgley, C. (2011) *2nd Annual Endodontic Board Review and Scientific Update*. College of Diplomates of the ABE and Columbia College of Dental Medicine, NY.

Simon, J.H., Chimenti, R.A. & Mintz, G.A. (1982) Clinical significance of the pulse granuloma. *Journal of Endodontics* **8**, 116–119.

Siqueira, J.F. Jr. & Rocas, I.N. (2005) Exploiting molecular methods to explore endodontic infections: Part 2 – Redefining the endodontic microbiota. *Journal of Endodontics* **31**, 488–498.

Souza, R.A. (2006) The importance of apical patency and cleaning of the apical foramen on root canal preparation. *Brazilian Dental Journal* **17**, 6–9.

Torabinejad, M., Kettering, J.D., McGraw, J.C. *et al.* (1988) Factors associated with endodontic interappointment emergencies of teeth with necrotic pulps. *Journal of Endodontics* **14**, 261–266.

Wolcott, J., Rossman, L.E. & Hasselgeren, G. (2011) Management of endodontic emergencies. *Cohen's Pathways of the Pulp* (eds. K. Hargreaves & S. Cohen), 10th edn, pp. 40–48. St. Louis, MO: Elsevier.

6

Emergency Case III:
Pulpal Debridement, Incision and Drainage (Extra-oral)

Amr Radwan and Katia Mattos

LEARNING OBJECTIVES
- To understand cases appropriate for incision and drainage.
- To understand the armamentarium for incision and drainage.
- To understand the various methods for performing incision and drainage.
- To understand the proper use of adjuncts during incision and drainage.

	Molars			Premolars		Canine	Incisors				Canine	Premolars		Molars		
							Maxillary arch									
Universal tooth designation system	1	2	3	4	5	6	7	8	9	10	11	12	13	14	15	16
International standards organization designation system	18	17	16	15	14	13	12	11	21	22	23	24	25	26	27	28
Palmer method	8⌋	7⌋	6⌋	5⌋	4⌋	3⌋	2⌋	1⌋	⌊1	⌊2	⌊3	⌊4	⌊5	⌊6	⌊7	⌊8
Palmer method	8⌉	7⌉	6⌉	5⌉	4⌉	3⌉	2⌉	1⌉	⌈1	⌈2	⌈3	⌈4	⌈5	⌈6	⌈7	⌈8
International standards organization designation system	48	47	46	45	44	43	42	41	31	32	33	34	35	36	37	38
Universal tooth designation system	32	31	30	29	28	27	26	25	24	23	22	21	20	19	18	17
							Mandibular arch									
		Right									**Left**					

Clinical Cases in Endodontics, First Edition. Edited by Takashi Komabayashi.
© 2018 John Wiley & Sons, Inc. Published 2018 by John Wiley & Sons, Inc.

Chief Complaint

"My lower right side is swollen, and I can barely open my mouth. My whole right side hurts so much."

Medical History

The patient (Pt) was a 43-year-old Caucasian male. Vital signs were as follows: Blood pressure (BP) 122/78 mmHg right arm seated (RAS), pulse 72 beats per minute (BPM) and regular, respiratory rate (RR) 18 breaths per minute, temperature (T) 99° F. A complete review of systems was conducted. There were no known drug allergies (NKDA).

The Pt was American Society of Anesthesiologists Physical Status Scale (ASA) Class I and reported no contraindications to dental treatment (Tx).

Dental History

The Pt presented for emergency Tx on his lower right side of his jaw. The Pt started experiencing severe pain on his lower right side two days prior, and he had not been able to sleep. Over the previous 48 hours, swelling had developed in the same area. His general dentist prescribed Augmentin® 250 mg three times daily (TID), and referred him for evaluation and Tx of tooth #31.

Clinical Evaluation
Examinations
Extra-oral Examination (EOE)

Facial swelling of the right submandibular area and facial asymmetry were noted (Figure 6.1). The swelling was about 5 × 4 cm and red in color. The skin was

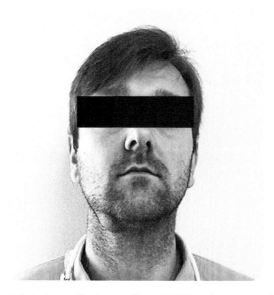

Figure 6.1 Submandibular swelling of LRQ and associated facial asymmetry.

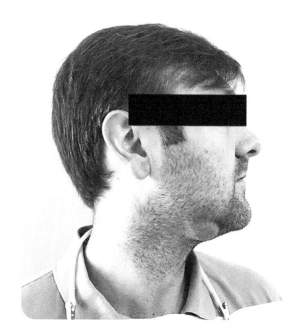

Figure 6.2 Skin is red with a shiny spot at the point of highest fluctuance.

warm on palpation with a shiny spot in the middle of the swelling (Figure 6.2). Moderate tenderness to palpation was noted on the soft tissue adjacent to tooth #31. Lymphadenopathy of the submandibular and neck areas was observed. Temporomandibular joint (TMJ) was asymptomatic with no popping, clicking, or deviation on opening.

Intra-oral Examination (IOE)

The Pt's oral hygiene was fair. There were no missing teeth. Periodontal pocket probing depths were all less than 3 mm on teeth #29, #30, and #31. All teeth responded normally to pulp sensibility tests except tooth #31, which did not respond to cold or electric pulp test and was tender to percussion and palpation. Tooth #31 showed class 2 mobility and a large carious lesion.

Diagnostic Tests

Tooth	#29	#30	#31
Percussion	−	−	++
Palpation	−	−	++
Cold	+	+	−
Mobility	1	1	2
EPT	36/80	38/80	80/80

EPT: Electric pulp test; ++: Response to percussion and palpation; +: Normal response to cold; −: No response to percussion, palpation and cold

Radiographic Findings

Periapical (PA) and bitewing radiographs were taken. Teeth #29, #30, and #31 were studied. Tooth #30 presented with a radiopaque occlusal restoration and calcification of the pulp chamber. Tooth #29 was within normal limits (WNL) with normal pulp space and periodontal ligaments. Tooth #31 showed a radiolucent carious lesion on the mesial (M) wall and a 3 × 4 mm periapical radiolucency (PARL) around the distal (D) root (Figures 6.3 and 6.4).

Multiple composite restorations were observed on the bitewing radiograph (Figure 6.5).

Pretreatment Diagnosis
Pulpal

Pulp Necrosis, tooth #31

Apical

Acute Apical Abscess, tooth #31

Treatment Plan
Recommended

Emergency: Incision and Drainage (I&D)
Definitive: Non-surgical root canal treatment (NSRCT) on tooth #31

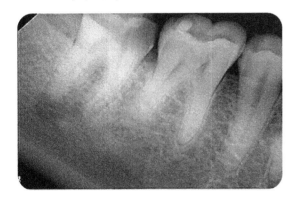

Figure 6.3 Preoperative periapical radiograph of tooth #31.

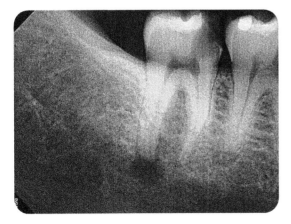

Figure 6.4 Preoperative periapical radiograph of tooth #31.

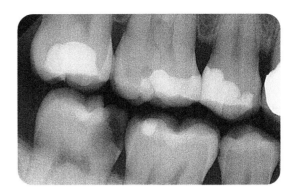

Figure 6.5 Preoperative bitewing radiograph of tooth #31.

Alternative

Extraction of tooth #31, no treatment

Restorative

Core build up and full coverage coronal restoration

Prognosis

Favorable	Questionable	Unfavorable
X		

Clinical Procedures: Treatment Record

First visit (Day 1): Reviewed medical history (RMHX). Vital signs were as follows: BP 122/78 mmHg RAS, pulse 72 BPM and regular, RR 18 breaths per minute. T was 99° F. All Tx options were reviewed with the Pt, including extraction. The Pt elected NSRCT and informed consent was obtained. Anesthesia was obtained by 72 mg of 2% lidocaine (lido) with 1:100,000 epinephrine (epi) (0.036 mg) administered via inferior alveolar nerve block (IANB) and via infiltration of the buccal (B) mucosa B of tooth #31.

Rubber dam isolation (RDI) was placed. Caries were excavated and access was prepared with a #4 round bur, using a high speed handpiece and copious water irrigation. The canals were identified using an endodontic explorer. The working length (WL) was determined by using a size-15 Lexicon® K-file (Dentsply Sirona, Johnson City, TN, USA), along with an electronic apex locator Root ZX®II (J. Morita, Kyoto, Japan). No drainage was observed through the canals. Canals were cleaned and shaped using Vortex Blue® nickel titanium (NiTi) rotary files (Dentsply Sirona, Johnson City, TN, USA). Irrigation of the canal system was performed with 10 ml of 6% sodium hypochlorite (NaOCl), following each instrument.

The canals were dried with premeasured medium and coarse paper points. Calcium hydroxide [Ca(OH)$_2$] (Ultracal® XS, Ultradent Products Inc., South Jordan, UT, USA) was applied as an interappointment, intracanal medicament. Cavit™ (3M, Two Harbors, MN, USA) was used as a temporary seal to the coronal access. The occlusion was examined and adjusted.

I&D procedure: The extra-oral operative area was disinfected with iodine tincture. The Pt was prepared and draped in the standard fashion for an extra-oral procedure. The area was shaved prior to the incision. A 3 cm horizontal incision was made in the most dependent area of the fluctuance. Peripheral pressure was applied towards the incision and a significant amount of purulent exudate was produced (Figure 6.6). The incision was irrigated with 5 ml of 0.9% sodium chloride (NaCl) solution. No drain was placed. The Pt was given a prescription for Amoxicillin 500 mg TID for infection and swelling, and ibuprofen 800 mg four times daily (QID) for pain.

Second visit (2-week follow-up): Pt returned two weeks later, asymptomatic (ASX).

RMHX. BP 123/76 mmHg, pulse was 71 BPM and regular. No swelling was observed. Extra-oral incision site showed normal color and texture with no swelling. 1 cm scar from the incision was observed (Figure 6.7). Anesthesia was obtained by 72 mg of 2% lidocaine with 1:100,000 epi (0.036 mg) administered via IANB and B infiltration of the mucosa of tooth #31.

A RDI was placed. The temporary restoration was removed. The canals were irrigated with 10 ml of 6% NaOCl, followed by 5 ml of 17% of Ethylenediaminetetraacetic acid (EDTA, Vista Dental Products Racine, WI, USA) and 3 ml of 2%

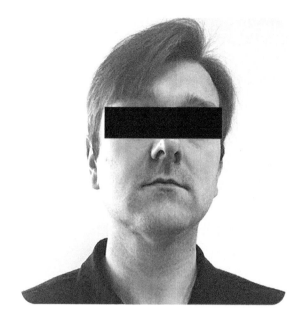

Figure 6.7 Two weeks after emergency I&D, patient returned asymptomatic. Skin does not appear red. No swelling noted. Small linear scar present at site of I&D.

chlorhexidine gluconate solution (CHX; Vista Dental Products) as a final irrigation. The canals were dried with paper points, then master cones were fitted and a radiograph was taken (Figure 6.8).

The canals were obturated with gutta-percha and AH Plus® Root Canal Sealer (Dentsply Sirona, Konstanz, Germany), using warm vertical compaction with Calamus® Dual (Dentsply Sirona, Johnson City, TN, USA). The floor of the pulp chamber was etched and bonded with Prime&Bond® XP (Dentsply Sirona, Konstanz, Germany). Flowable composite (Ultradent, South Jordan, UT, USA) was placed on the obturated canal orifice. A sterile cotton and Cavit™ were used as a temporary seal to the coronal access. The occlusion

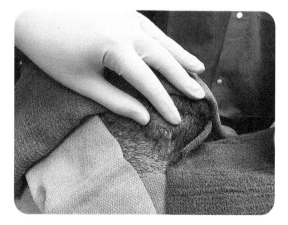

Figure 6.6 I&D performed, abundant purulent discharge produced. Area and patient isolated with standard draping.

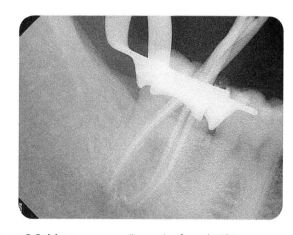

Figure 6.8 Master cone radiograph of tooth #31.

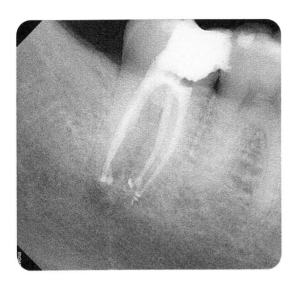

Figure 6.9 Postoperative radiograph of tooth #31.

was examined and adjusted. A postoperative radiograph was taken of tooth #31 (Figure 6.9). Postoperative instructions (POI) were given to the Pt. The Pt was

referred back to his dentist for permanent restoration of tooth #31 and continuation of his Tx plan.

Working length, apical size, and obturation technique

Canal	Working Length	Apical Size, Taper	Obturation Materials and Techniques
MB	19.5 mm	30, .04	AH Plus® sealer, Vertical compaction
ML	19.5 mm	30, .04	AH Plus® sealer, Vertical compaction
DB	19.0 mm	40, .04	AH Plus® sealer, Vertical compaction
DL	19.5 mm	40, .04	AH Plus® sealer, Vertical compaction

Post-Treatment Evaluations

The Pt was scheduled for a postoperative evaluation after six months and one year to evaluate the coronal restoration and healing of the periapical lesion.

Self-Study Questions

A. What are the diagnostic criteria for performing I&D?

B. What are the advantages of I&D?

C. What are the main principles of I&D?

D. What are the main adjuncts to performing I&D?

E. Describe the armamentarium for I&D.

F. Which are the fascial spaces of the head and neck?

Answers to Self-Study Questions

A. A patient presenting with swelling can have multiple manifestations. The swelling may be fluctuant or firm. It can also be localized or diffuse, also referred to as cellulitis. Localized swellings are confined within the oral cavity, whereas cellulitis can spread to adjacent soft tissues along fascial planes (Natkin 1974; Sandor *et al.* 1998). Incision and drainage is indicated when soft tissue swelling is present and drainage through the canal system cannot be achieved. I&D is most effective when the swelling is localized, soft and fluctuant (Frank *et al.* 1983).

B. Incision and drainage allows for decompression of the edematous tissues and provides significant pain relief for the patient. I&D also prevents further spread of infection through fascial planes and muscle attachments. I&D provides a portal for irrigation and placement of the drain. During I&D, a pathway is created for bacterial by-products, as well as inflammatory mediators (Wolcott, Rossman & Hasselgeren 2011). However, I&D allows for the collection of samples for culturing the offending microorganisms. More importantly, I&D will alter the chemical environment to one that is more aerobic, thus less optimal for the more virulent anaerobic bacteria.

C. The main principles for performing I&D are:
- A stab incision needs to be made through the periosteum, at the point of greatest fluctuance.
- The incision should be parallel to the blood vessels.
- The incision should avoid any vital structures (Siqueira & Rocas 2011).
- The incision should be made on healthy skin or mucosa, as incising areas manifesting breakdown, such as a sinus tract, will delay healing and may lead to scar formation.
- All areas of the abscess cavity should be explored, allowing for compartmentalized areas to be evacuated.
- Warm saltwater rinses should be used to keep the incision site clean, and also to increase blood flow to the area, intensifying host defenses (Harrington & Natkin 1992).

D. No pain medication or antibiotic can replace the role of debridement of the root canal system or of I&D of the associated soft tissues. However, both classes of medications are important adjuncts that can be used to provide more rapid and consistent relief to the patient.

The prescription of antibiotics should always be judicious and reserved for patients presenting systemic involvement. Symptoms such as high fever, trismus, and malaise warrant the prescription of antibiotics. Patients who show signs of progressive infection when all above-mentioned interventions have been performed or immunocompromised patients are also indicated for antibiotic treatment (Harrington & Natkin 1992; Sandor *et al.* 1998).

NSAIDs, and especially ibuprofen, are the drug of choice for acute dental pain. Because of their anti-inflammatory effect, NSAIDs can suppress swelling and have analgesic and antipyretic properties.

E. The instrument tray for I&D should hold:
- Aspirating syringe for local anesthesia
- #15 blade and blade holder
- Curved and/or straight mosquito hemostat
- Gauze director
- Needle holder, suture material, and scissors
- One-quarter inch Penrose drain
- Culture bottle and/or a syringe to aspirate pus to send for culture
- Gauze dressing, bandage, tape, etc.
- Skin scrub preparation, alcohol sponge, disinfectant

F. A case presenting with swelling can develop into a life-threatening medical emergency. Depending on the location of the apices of the infected tooth as it relates to the muscular attachments, the swelling can be localized or it can extend into a fascial space.

An odontogenic infection can spread through these potential anatomic areas:

- Mandible and below (buccal vestibule, body of mandible, mental space, submental space, sublingual space, submandibular space)
- Cheek and lateral face (buccal vestibule, buccal space, submasseteric space, temporal space)
- Pharyngeal and cervical areas (pterygomandibular, parapharyngeal, cervical)

- Midface (palate, base of upper lip, canine spaces, periorbital spaces) (Hohl et al. 1983)

Any swelling involving the submental, sublingual, and submandibular spaces is diagnosed as Ludwig's angina. These cases should be immediately referred to the hospital, ER, or an on-call oral surgeon, as they can advance into the pharyngeal and cervical spaces, obstructing the patient's airway.

References

Frank, A. L., Simon, J. S., Abou-Rass, M. et al. (1983) Surgical procedures. Clinical and Surgical Endodontics: Concepts in Practice (eds. A.L. Frank, J.S. Simon, M. Frank et al.), pp. 91–92. Philadelphia: J.P. Lippincott.

Harrington, G. W. & Natkin, E. (1992) Midtreatment flare-ups. Dental Clinics of North America **36**, 409–423.

Hohl, T. H., Whitacre, R. J., Hooley, J. R. et al. (1983) A Self-Instructional Guide: Diagnosis and Treatment of Odontogenic Infections. Seattle, WA: Stoma Press.

Natkin, E. (1974) Treatment of endodontic emergencies. Dental Clinics of North America **18**, 243–255.

Sandor, G. K., Low, D. E., Judd, P. L. et al. (1998) Antimicrobial treatment options in the management of odontogenic infections. Journal of the Canadian Dental Association **64**, 508–514.

Siqueira, J. F. & Rocas, I. (2011) Microbiology and treatment of endodontic infections. In: Cohen's Pathways of the Pulp (eds. K. Hargreaves & S. Cohen), 10th edn, pp. 559–600. St. Louis, MO: Mosby Elsevier.

Wolcott, J. Rossman, L. E. & Hasselgeren, G. (2011) Management of endodontic emergencies. In: Cohen's Pathways of the Pulp (eds. K. Hargreaves & S. Cohen), 10th edn, pp. 40–48. St. Louis, MO: Elsevier.

7

Non-surgical Root Canal Treatment Case I: Maxillary Anterior

Denise Foran

LEARNING OBJECTIVES

- To describe anatomic variations of the maxillary anterior teeth.
- To understand the elements of performing a clinical endodontic workup in the maxillary anterior region.
- To understand how to conduct an appropriate radiological examination of the maxillary anterior region.
- To understand how to perform endodontic therapy on a maxillary incisor.
- To discuss how cone beam-computed tomography (CBCT) can be useful in the diagnosis and treatment of the maxillary anterior teeth.

	Molars			Premolars		Canine	Incisors				Canine	Premolars		Molars		
							Maxillary arch									
Universal tooth designation system	1	2	3	4	5	6	7	8	9	10	11	12	13	14	15	16
International standards organization designation system	18	17	16	15	14	13	12	11	21	22	23	24	25	26	27	28
Palmer method	8	7	6	5	4	3	2	1	1	2	3	4	5	6	7	8
Palmer method	8	7	6	5	4	3	2	1	1	2	3	4	5	6	7	8
International standards organization designation system	48	47	46	45	44	43	42	41	31	32	33	34	35	36	37	38
Universal tooth designation system	32	31	30	29	28	27	26	25	24	23	22	21	20	19	18	17
							Mandibular arch									
	Right								**Left**							

Clinical Cases in Endodontics, First Edition. Edited by Takashi Komabayashi.
© 2018 John Wiley & Sons, Inc. Published 2018 by John Wiley & Sons, Inc.

Chief Complaint

"I have many fillings in my front teeth and one of them towards the left feels like it is loose."

Medical History

The patient (Pt) was a 34-year old Caucasian female. A complete review of systems was conducted. Vital signs were recorded: Blood pressure (BP) was 110/72 mmHg, respiratory rate (RR) 16 breaths per minute, pulse 70 beats per minute (BPM). The Pt denied any surgical history (Hx). She reported an allergy to Levaquin®. She was taking Klonopin® 0.5 mg every 12 hours (Q12H) for generalized anxiety disorder and paroxetine 20 mg daily (QD) for depression. She denied alcohol and drug abuse and was a non-smoker.

Pt was classified as American Society of Anesthesiologists Physical Scale Status (ASA) Class II.

Dental History

The Pt reported that her dentist restored a few cavities on her front teeth about a year ago. She did not have any discomfort prior to the treatment (Tx). About a year after the restorations were made, she stated that one of her teeth felt weak and was starting to change color. She reported that she had orthodontic therapy as a teenager but has never had any major dental problems.

Clinical Evaluation (Diagnostic Procedures)

Examinations

Extra-oral Examination (EOE)

EOE was within normal limits (WNL). Skin and perioral regions were normal in color and texture. Temporomandibular joint (TMJ) was WNL. There was no evidence of clicking or popping or signs of any dislocation. Maximal opening was WNL. There was no lymphadenopathy of the head and neck regions upon palpation.

Intra-oral Examination (IOE)

IOE of the soft tissues was WNL. Gingival tissues were normal in color and texture. Oral cancer screening was negative and oral hygiene was good. Periodontal probings measured 3 mm on all surfaces of the maxillary anterior teeth. There was no bleeding on probing and no gingival recession. IOE exam of the hard tissues revealed a complete adult dentition and multiple composite restorations on the maxillary anterior teeth. The Pt had a Class I molar occlusion.

Diagnostic Tests

Tooth	#9	#10	#11
Percussion	−	−	−
Palpation	−	−	−
Cold	+	−	+
EPT	+	−	+

EPT: Electric pulp test; + : Normal response; − : No response

Radiographic Findings

One periapical (PA) radiograph was taken (Figure 7.1). Tooth #8 was restored with a distal (D) composite restoration. Teeth #9 and #10 were restored with mesial (M) and D composite restorations. Tooth #11 did not appear to have any restorations. There was a periapical radiolucency at the root apex of tooth #10. All other teeth had normal periapices.

Pretreatment Diagnosis
Pulpal

Pulp Necrosis, tooth #10

Apical

Asymptomatic Apical Periodontitis, tooth #10

Treatment Plan
Recommended

Emergency: None
Definitive: Non-surgical Root Canal Therapy (NSRCT) of tooth #10

Alternative

Extraction, no treatment

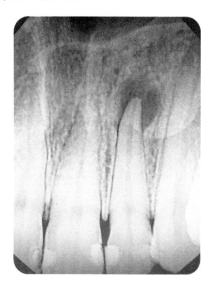

Figure 7.1 Preoperative radiograph of tooth #10.

Restorative

Porcelain crown

Prognosis

Favorable	Questionable	Unfavorable
X		

Clinical Procedures: Treatment Record

First visit (Day 1): Informed consent was obtained for NSRCT of tooth #10. Local anesthesia was achieved via local infiltration in the buccal (B) mucosa overlying tooth #10 with 34 mg of lidocaine (lido) and 0.017mg of epinephrine (epi). Tooth isolation was achieved with a 9A clamp on tooth #10 and a rubber dam (RD) with frame. Initial access was made through the lingual surface (L) of tooth #10 with a FG #4 SL round bur and a high speed handpiece. The access cavity was examined with an operating microscope to investigate the presence of any additional canals. A size-15 Lexicon® K-file (Dentsply Sirona, Johnson City, TN, USA) was placed into the canal, and the working length (WL) was determined with the use of an electronic apex locator (Root ZX®II, J. Morita, Kyoto, Japan). The WL was determined to be 23 mm from the incisal edge of tooth #10. The canal was instrumented using size #15, #20 and #25 ReadySteel® FlexoFiles® (Dentsply Sirona, Ballaigues, Switzerland) and rotary files (Dentsply Sirona). Rotary instrumentation was achieved with the use of a crown down technique to a master apical file of size #35. The canal was irrigated with 6.0 ml of 5.25% sodium hypochlorite (NaOCl) throughout the instrumentation process. The canal was dried with sterile paper points. Inter-appointment medicament of Ca(OH)$_2$ paste was placed in canal (Ultradent, South Jordan, UT, USA). The tooth was temporized with a cotton pellet and Cavit™ G (3M, Two Harbors, MN, USA). Occlusion was adjusted for Pt comfort. Post-operative instructions (POI) were given. The Pt was advised to take over-the-counter (OTC) ibuprofen 600 mg every 6 hours as needed for (PRN) pain. The Pt was advised to contact the office if she experienced any severe pain or swelling. An appointment was scheduled for the completion of endodontic treatment (Tx).

Second visit (Day 7): The Pt returned after one week for the completion of endodontic treatment. She reported no complications since the initial Tx visit. Local anesthesia was achieved via local infiltration in buccal (B) mucosa overlying tooth #10 with 34 mg of lido and 0.018 mg of epi. Dental dam isolation was

accomplished using protocol from first visit. The temporary filling was removed and the canal was irrigated with 6.0 ml of 5.25% NaOCl, 1.0 cc of 17% Ethylenediaminetetraacetic acid (EDTA) and 3.0 ml of 2% chlorhexidine. A master cone, size #35/.04 gutta-percha point (Dentsply Sirona, Petropolis, Brazil) was placed to proper length with tug-back. A radiograph was taken to confirm placement of the master cone (Figure 7.2). The tooth was obturated using lateral condensation technique and zinc oxide eugenol-based sealer (Roth International, Chicago, IL, USA). Tooth #10 was temporized with a cotton pellet and Cavit™ G. A final post-treatment radiograph was taken (Figure 7.3). The Pt was referred to her general dentist for a permanent restoration. She was placed on a one-year endodontic

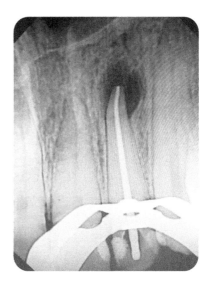

Figure 7.2 Master cone radiograph of tooth #10.

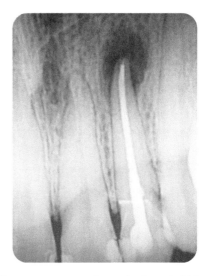

Figure 7.3 Post-treatment radiograph of tooth #10.

recall to evaluate periapical healing. A post-operative (PO) report was sent to her general dentist.

Working length, apical size, and obturation technique

Canal	Working Length	Apical Size, Taper	Obturation Materials and Techniques
Single	23.0 mm	35, .04	Zinc oxide eugenol sealer, Lateral condensation

Post-Treatment Evaluations

Third visit (1-year follow-up): The Pt returned for PO Tx evaluation of tooth #10. The Pt had remained asymptomatic and her chief complaint had resolved. The soft tissue was WNL and periodontal probing's were WNL and unchanged. One PA radiograph was taken. There was evidence of PA healing of the initial radiolucency associated with the periapex of tooth #10 (Figure 7.4). The tooth had been restored with a

permanent bonded core as per the general dentist. Teeth #9 and #11 were stable.

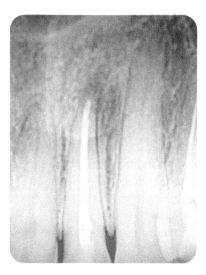

Figure 7.4 One-year post-treatment radiograph of tooth #10.

Self-Study Questions

A. What anatomic structure should be taken into consideration when radiographically evaluating maxillary anterior teeth?

B. How should diagnostic testing be performed in the maxillary anterior region?

C. What kind of initial radiographic exam is appropriate for an endodontic work up in the maxillary anterior region?

D. What is an example of an anatomical variation associated with the maxillary anterior teeth that can affect non-surgical endodontic therapy?

E. What is an example of a developmental anomaly associated with the maxillary anterior teeth that can affect non-surgical endodontic therapy?

Answers to Self-Study Questions

A. Failure to recognize normal anatomy of the anterior maxilla may result in an incorrect diagnosis. The nasopalatine canal, also called the incisive canal or anterior palatine canal, has been described as a canal located in the middle of the palate, just posterior to the roots of central maxillary incisors (Figure 7.5). The opening of this canal can appear as an oval-shaped radiolucency and must not be mistaken for a periapical radiolucency (PARL). A true PARL will be associated with tooth attachment. The radiolucent periodontal ligament (PDL) space should be evaluated carefully for any thickening and discontinuation. A change in the width and/or shape of the PDL aids in the diagnosis of periapical pathosis (PAP) (Strindberg 1956).

B. Diagnostic testing for disease of endodontic origin includes thermal testing, electric pulp testing percussion, and palpation. In the maxillary anterior there are systematic approaches to performing these tests (Figures 7.6, 7.7 and 7.8). Cold testing is a valuable and reliable tool to determine pulpal nerve status of permanent teeth

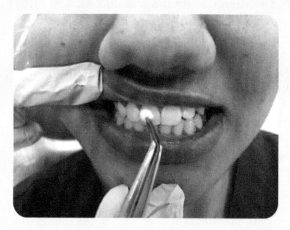

Figure 7.6 Cold testing using a cotton pellet saturated with ice refrigerant.

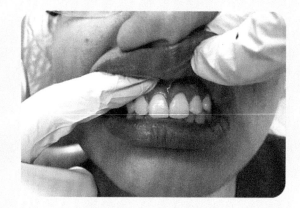

Figure 7.7 Digital palpation of apical mucosa.

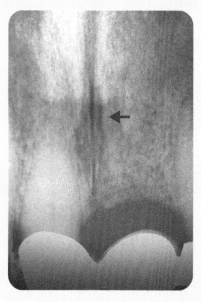

Figure 7.5 Nasopalatine foramen can be mistaken for an endodontic lesion.

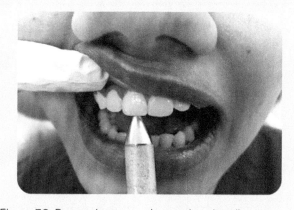

Figure 7.8 Percussion test using a mirror handle.

(Petersson *et al.* 1999). Electric pulp testing activates low threshold A-delta fibers and an ionic fluid shift that elicits a positive pulpal response in healthy pulps (Närhi *et al.* 1979). Percussion and palpation testing will give the clinician information regarding the status of the apical periodontal ligament. A significant cause of mechanical allodynia is inflammation of vital pulp tissue. This inflammation contributes to early stages of odontogenic pain (Owatz *et al.* 2007).

C. Endodontic therapy requires a radiographic exam in addition to clinical examination. Multiple periapical radiographs taken at different angulation have been shown to increase the accuracy of interpretation (Brynolf 1970). The natural curvature of the arch may cause the roots of the teeth to become superimposed. Different angulation will change position of the teeth on the image (Figures 7.9 and 7.10).

D. Maxillary anterior teeth typically have one root and one root canal (Vertucci 1984). However, there have been case reports of maxillary anterior teeth with two roots. Additional roots are not always visible on PA radiographs and are only discovered after endodontic access (Figure 7.11). The use of an endodontic operating microscope and/or CBCT may be useful in determining the presence of

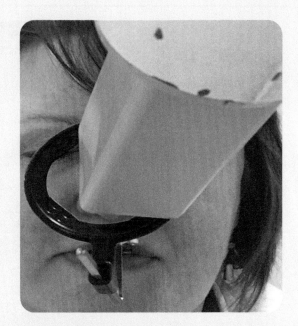

Figure 7.10 Different angulations for anterior periapical radiograph.

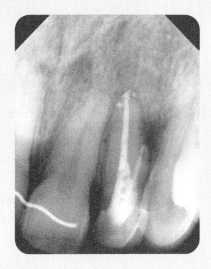

Figure 7.11 A radiograph of maxillary lateral incisor with two canals.

atypical anatomy (Patel *et al.* 2015). CBCT can also give the clinician more information on the extent of lesions. In Figure 7.12, one can appreciate a 3-D view of a periapical lesion and its relation to the buccal and palatal bone.

E. Dens invaginatus (DI) is a developmental anomaly resulting from the folding of the enamel organ into the dental papilla prior to calcification of dental tissues (Oehlers 1957; Gound 1997). The frequency of DI is reported to

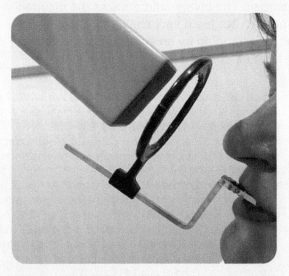

Figure 7.9 Paralleling technique for anterior periapical radiograph.

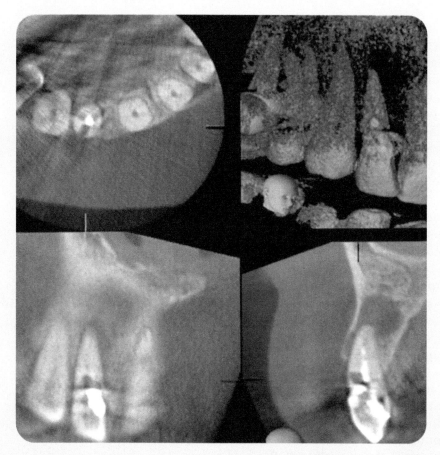

Figure 7.12 CBCT of maxillary right lateral incisor. The image on the upper left is a coronal view of an endodontically treated tooth #7. One can see a break in the buccal plate due to the resorptive defect. The image on the upper right is a 3-D creation of the maxilla. The images on lower right and lower left are sagittal and axial views of tooth #7, respectively. These views give the clinician information on the dimensions and extent of the lesion.

be 0.04–10%; its prevalence is the greatest in permanent lateral incisors (Gound 1997). A tooth with this anomaly is susceptible to pulp necrosis. The invagination makes the disinfection of these teeth very challenging and would be best handled by an endodontic specialist.

References

Brynolf, I. (1970) Roentgenolgic periapical diagnosis. IV. When is one roentgenogram not sufficient? *Swedish Dental Journal* **63**, 415–423.

Gound, T. G. (1997) Dens invaginatus – a pathway to pulpal pathology: A literature review. *Practical Periodontics and Aesthetic Dentistry* **9**, 585–594.

Närhi, M., Virtanen, A., Kuhta, J. *et al.* (1979) Electrical stimulation of teeth with a pulp tester in the cat. *Scandinavian Journal of Dental Research* **87**, 32–38.

Oehlers, F. A. (1957) Dens invaginatus (dilated composite odontome). I. Variations of the invagination process and associated anterior crown forms. *Oral Surgery, Oral Medicine, and Oral Pathology* **10**, 1204–1218.

Owatz, C. B., Khan, A. A., Schindler, W. G. *et al.* (2007) The incidence of mechanical allodynia in patients with irreversible pulpitis. *Journal of Endodontics* **33**, 552–556.

Patel, S., Durack, C., Abella, F. *et al.* (2015) Cone beam computed tomography in Endodontics – a review. *International Endodontic Journal* **48**, 3–15.

Petersson, K., Söderström, C., Kiani-Anaraki, M. *et al.* (1999) Evaluation of the ability of thermal and electrical tests to register pulp vitality. *Endodontics & Dental Traumatology* **15**, 127–131.

Strindberg, L. Z. (1956) The dependence of the results of pulp therapy on certain factors. An analytic study based on radiographic and clinical follow-up examinations. *Acta Odontologica Scandinavica* **14** (Suppl. 21).

Vertucci, F. J. (1984) Root canal anatomy of the human permanent teeth. *Oral Surgery, Oral Medicine, and Oral Pathology* **58**, 589–599.

8

Non-surgical Root Canal Treatment Case II: Mandibular Anterior

Jessica Russo Revand and John M. Russo

LEARNING OBJECTIVES
- To understand the particular challenges posed by endodontic treatment of mandibular incisors and optimal clinical techniques.
- To understand the morphologic types of root canal anatomy in mandibular incisors.
- To understand the reasons for the access preparation outline on mandibular incisors and when to alter the design.
- To understand the various techniques for identifying and uncovering complex anatomy in mandibular incisors.
- To understand the odontogenic and non-odontogenic causes of periapical radiolucencies in the anterior mandible and importance of vitality testing.

Clinical Cases in Endodontics, First Edition. Edited by Takashi Komabayashi.
© 2018 John Wiley & Sons, Inc. Published 2018 by John Wiley & Sons, Inc.

Chief Complaint

"My tooth hurts and my gums are swollen."

Medical History

The patient (Pt) was a 12-year-old male. Review of systems indicated cardiovascular, within normal limits (WNL); respiratory, WNL; gastrointestinal, WNL; genitourinary, WNL; musculoskeletal, WNL; neurologic, WNL; endocrine, WNL. There were no current medications and no known drug allergies (NKDA). Vital signs were as follows: Blood pressure (BP) = 94/60 mmHg left arm seated (LAS); pulse = 92 beats per minute (BPM).

The Pt was considered American Society of Anesthesiologists Physical Status Scale (ASA) Class I.

Dental History

Complete maxillary and mandibular orthodontic treatment was initiated six months prior to his initial endodontic visit. Pt's parents reported a history of trauma to the lower anteriors approximately two years prior to placement of orthodontic brackets. He began to experience pain and swelling in the area of tooth #25 approximately one week ago with some relief when drainage occurred through a sinus tract the day before.

Clinical Evaluation (Diagnostic Procedures)
Examinations
Extra-oral Examination (EOE)

No lymphadenopathy was present and the Pt was afebrile.

Intra-oral examination (IOE)

Swelling of the buccal (B) mucosa appeared in the area of the right mandibular incisors with a sinus tract on the B gingiva between teeth #25 and #26 (Figure 8.1). Probing of tooth #25 from mesial (M) to distal (D) of Facial (3 mm, 2 mm and 3 mm) and M to D of Lingual (3 mm, 2 mm and 3 mm).

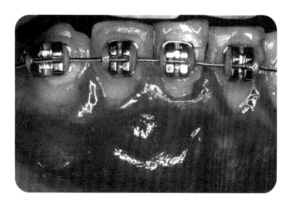

Figure 8.1 Preoperative buccal swelling with sinus tract between teeth #25 and 26. (Photograph courtesy of Dr. Domenico Ricucci).

Diagnostic Tests

Tooth	#24	#25	#26
Percussion	−	++	−
Palpation	−	+	−
Cold	+	-	+
Mobility	0	2	0
EPT	+	-	+
Sinus Tract	No	Yes	No

EPT: Electric pulp test, ++: Exaggerated response, +: Response to percussion or palpation, and normal response to cold and EPT; -: No response to percussion, palpation, cold, or EPT

Radiographic Findings

The periapical (PA) radiograph showed the lower mandibular teeth #23–#27 (Figure 8.2). The teeth were non-carious and had orthodontic brackets and wire present. Normal bone height was present. There was a periapical radiolucency (PARL) at the apex of tooth #25 approximately 4 mm x 6 mm that extended along the distal (D) surface of tooth #25 to just below the crestal bone. The apex of tooth #25 appeared to be slightly mesially displaced.

Pre-Treatment Diagnosis
Pulpal

Pulp Necrosis, tooth #25

Apical

Chronic Apical Abscess, tooth #25

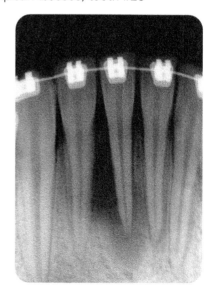

Figure 8.2 Preoperative radiograph of teeth #23–27. Note the slight mesial displacement of the apex of tooth #25 and bone loss along the distal root surface. (Radiograph courtesy of Dr. Domenico Ricucci).

Treatment Plan
Recommended

Emergency: Pulp debridement with calcium hydroxide (Ca(OH)₂)

Definitive: Non-surgical root canal treatment (NSRCT)

Alternative

No treatment, extraction

Restorative

Composite core build-up

Prognosis

Favorable	Questionable	Unfavorable
X		

Clinical Procedures: Treatment Record

First visit (Day 1): BP was 94/60 mmHg LAS, pulse was 92 BPM. After clinical and radiographic examination, diagnosis, and treatment (Tx) planning, the risks and benefits of Tx were discussed with the Pt and his parents. Informed consent for endodontic Tx was obtained from Pt's parents. Anesthesia was achieved by topical 20% benzocaine followed by administration of mental nerve block, B and lingual (L) infiltration with 36 mg lidocaine (lido) with 0.018 mg epinephrine (epi). Rubber dam isolation (RDI) was achieved with Ivory® 9 clamp (Heraeus Kulzer, Wehrheim, Germany) placed apically to the orthodontic bracket and wire on tooth #25. The coronal surface was wiped with a cotton pellet soaked in 3% sodium hypochlorite (NaOCl). The access cavity was prepared with #2 surgical length round bur and fissure bur on a high speed handpiece. The outline of the endodontic access was shaped as an oval with the incisal edge slightly flared to aid in visualization of the canal orifice (Figure 8.3). The area of the cingulum was extended towards the L to aid in the detection of a possible L canal. After the B canal was identified, the L canal was detected by angling the tip of the size #10 K-file by 30° and running the tip of the file along the L surface of the B canal. Working lengths (WL) were determined with radiographs and the use of an electronic apex locator Root ZX® II (J. Morita, Kyoto, Japan)using a size #10 K-file (Figure 8.4). The two canals were found to be confluent in the apical third (Vertucci type II configuration). The canals were instrumented manually with K-type and Hedstrom files in the apical third to a size #20 Hedstrom file and with Gates Glidden burs #2, #3, and #4 in the coronal two-thirds of

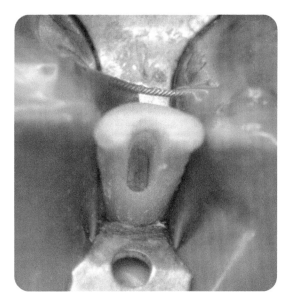

Figure 8.3 Access opening tooth #25 after obturation completed. The preparation has been extended half-way through the incisal edge to improve access to the large canal space in a young patient. The mesio-distal preparation is conservative to reflect the external and internal anatomy. (Photograph courtesy of Dr. Domenico Ricucci).

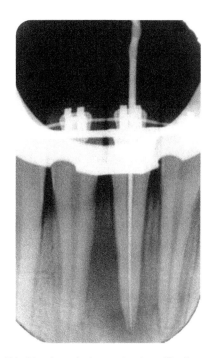

Figure 8.4 Working-length determination. (Radiograph courtesy of Dr. Domenico Ricucci).

each canal. Irrigating solution was 1% NaOCl. The canals were dried with sterile paper points. Ca(OH)₂ paste was placed in the canal with a Lentulo® Spiral Filler (Dentsply Sirona, Ballaigues, Switzerland) and condensed with paper points and cotton pellet. The access cavity was sealed with Cavit™ (3M, Two Harbors, MN, USA). Post-operative instructions (POI) given including the use of warm salt water rinses to encourage drainage of the swelling through the sinus tract.

Second visit (Day 8): The Pt was asymptomatic and the sinus tract had closed. There was no evidence of soft tissue swelling in the facial vestibule of teeth #24–#26. Oral consent obtained from Pt's parents for Tx. Anesthesia was achieved by topical 20% benzocaine followed by administration of mental nerve block, B and L infiltration with 36 mg lido with 0.018 mg epi. RDI was achieved with Ivory 9 clamp placed apically to the orthodontic bracket and wire on tooth #25. The instrumentation was completed to apical size #40 Hedstrom file with step-back hand instrumentation to size #60 using K-type and Hedstrom files. Irrigating solution was 1% NaOCl. The canals were dried with sterile paper points. A size #40 gutta-percha (GP) point was placed in the B canal (to the WL) and size #30 GP point in the L canal (to the level of confluence) with Pulp Canal Sealer™ Extended Working Time (EWT) sealer (Kerr Corporation, Romulus, MI). The canals were obturated with cold lateral compaction using the blue finger spreader and fine–fine accessory points. Excess GP was removed to the level of the cementoenamel junction (CEJ) using a heated spoon excavator. A permanent core build-up was placed using etch, bonding agent, and composite. The composite surface was polished and the occlusion checked. POI were given to the Pt and his parents. A postoperative (PO) radiograph showed sealer extrusion through a large L canal on the D root surface (Figures 8.5 and 8.6).

Working length, apical size, and obturation technique

Canal	Working Length	Apical Size	Obturation Materials and Techniques
B	22.0 mm	40	Pulp Canal Sealer™ EWT, Cold lateral compaction
L	22.0 mm	40	Pulp Canal Sealer™ EWT, Cold lateral compaction

Post-Treatment Evaluation

Third visit (13-year follow-up): A 13-year follow-up showed complete healing of the preoperative radiolucency with formation of a lamina dura along the entire root perimeter (Figure 8.7). Resorption of the extruded sealer on the D root surface was noted. Tooth

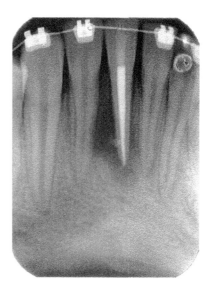

Figure 8.5 Postoperative radiograph of tooth #25. Oburation of the canal space includes fill of large lateral canal on the distal surface. (Radiograph courtesy of Dr. Domenico Ricucci).

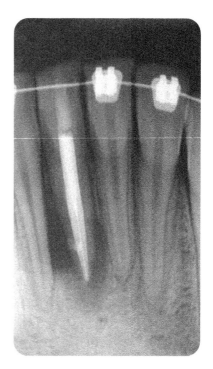

Figure 8.6 Postoperative angled radiograph to visualize complete obturation of the buccal and lingual canals. (Radiograph courtesy of Dr. Domenico Ricucci).

#25 was asymptomatic to percussion and palpation. There was 0 mobility on tooth #25. Probing depth was 3 mm, 2 mm and 3 mm (from M to D of Facial) and 3 mm, 2 mm and 3 mm (from M to D of Lingual).

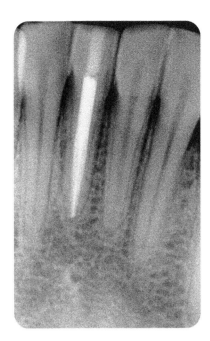

Figure 8.7 Thirteen-year follow-up. There is complete healing of the preoperative radiolucency and resorption of the extruded sealer on the distal surface of the root. (Radiograph courtesy of Dr. Domenico Ricucci).

Fourth visit (14-year follow-up): A 14-year follow up shows normal periapical tissues radiographically

(Figure 8.8). Tooth #25 was asymptomatic to percussion and palpation. There was 0 mobility on tooth #25. Probing depth was 3 mm, 2 mm and 3 mm (from M to D of Facial) and 3 mm, 2 mm and 3 mm (from M to D of Lingual).

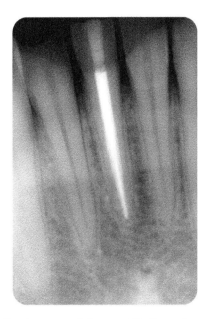

Figure 8.8 Fourteen-year follow-up. (Radiograph courtesy of Dr. Domenico Ricucci).

Self-Study Questions

A. What percentage of mandibular incisors have a second canal? What anatomic characteristics of mandibular incisors require special consideration?

B. What are the anatomic considerations when designing the access preparation for a mandibular incisor?

C. What instruments are useful when looking for a second canal on mandibular incisors?

D. How does one determine if a radiographic radiolucency is endodontic in origin or non-odontogenic?

E. What is the best restoration for the endodontically treated mandibular incisor?

Answers to Self-Study Questions

A. While mandibular incisors are typically single rooted teeth, the prevalence of two canals is relatively high. A small percentage of these teeth have two distinct roots. The complex root canal anatomy of mandibular incisors versus their maxillary counterparts is repeatedly confirmed in the literature (Table 8.1). As such, all mandibular central and lateral incisors should be approached as having two canals until proven otherwise.

The operator is encouraged to take angled radiographs preoperatively and during treatment for the purpose of identifying additional anatomy (Figure 8.9). Alternatively, the cone beam-computed tomography (CBCT) scan can clearly show the propensity for mandibular incisors to harbor two canals or even two roots (Figure 8.10) (Paes da Silva Ramos Fernandes *et al.* 2014). The prevalence of mandibular canines having two roots is the highest among mandibular incisors with the percentage reported as high as 12% (Rahimi *et al.* 2013).

B. As with all endodontic cases, the access preparation is the most important step in treatment of mandibular incisors. The entrance to the second canal on these mandibular incisors is lingual to the more easily located labial canal; hence proper access preparation is crucial to locate both canals. Ideal straight-line access to the apical foramen on the central and lateral incisors is topographically located at or labial to the incisal edge. A labial access preparation would also conserve more coronal dentin (Logani *et al.* 2009). For aesthetic reasons, however, the standard clinical access is through the center of

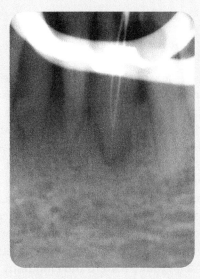

Figure 8.9 Angled working-length radiograph to aid in visualization of the second canal. (Radiograph courtesy of Dr. Domenico Ricucci).

Table 8.1 Root canal anatomy of mandibular incisors.

Author	Year	Number of Teeth	Tooth Type	One Coronal Canal	Two Coronal Canals	One Apical Foramen	Two Apical Foramina
Vertucci	1984	100	Central	70%	30%	97%	3%
		100	Lateral	75%	25%	98%	2%
Caliskan	1995	100	Central	69%	29%	96%	2%
		100	Lateral	69%	31%	98%	2%
		100	Canine	89%	11%	97%	3%
Rahimi	2013	186	Central	81%	19%	99.5%	0.5%
		128	Lateral	83%	17%	99.2%	0.8%
		131	Canine	93%	6%	100%	0%
Shaikh	2014	100	Lateral	61%	39%		
Lin	2014	706	Central	89%	11%		
		706	Lateral	74.5%	25.5%		

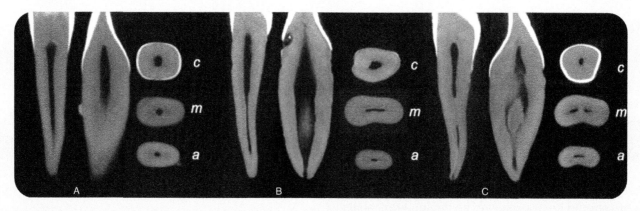

Figure 8.10 Micro-CT images of three different teeth to show the varying anatomic patterns: A: Vertucci type I with round canal, B: Vertucci type I with oval canal, C: Vertucci type III. Cross section images labeled as: c = cervical, m = middle, a = apical. (Image adapted from Paes da Silva Ramos Fernandes *et al.* (2014)).

the lingual surface of the tooth. Proper access preparation for mandibular incisors is depicted in Figure 8.11. Of note is the triangular outline on the central and lateral incisors to include the pulp horns. This important step will prevent future coronal discoloration due to pulp tissue left behind. The access shape may revert to oval in patients over the age of 40 as a result of the deposition of secondary dentin in the pulp chamber facilitating the conservation of coronal dentin (Nielsen & Shamohammadi 2005). It is important to extend the preparation both incisally and lingually toward the cingulum in all incisor teeth. It is the incisal extension that affords a

straight-line instrument access to the apical foramen and the lingual extension along the cingulum that provides the operator visualization of the lingual canal orifice (Figure 8.12). Given the relatively high percentages of two canals in these teeth, radiographic imaging with varied horizontal angulation is recommended to determine the presence or absence of a second canal (Mahajan *et al.* 2016). Of course, if CBCT imaging was available, it would be the most definitive means of determining the root canal anatomy. Once the access preparation is properly oriented and extended, the case becomes more predictably treatable.

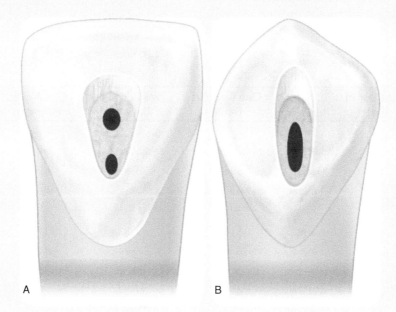

Figure 8.11 Access outline for A: the mandibular central and lateral incisors and B: the mandibular canine. (Illustration by Mr. Oran Suta.)

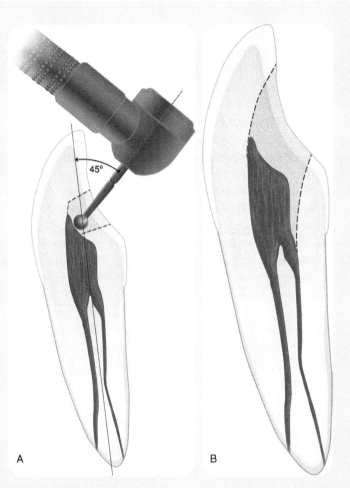

Figure 8.12 Lateral view of mandibular incisor showing A: Initial penetration with round bur until the pulp chamber is reached, B: Extension of the access prep towards the incisal edge and the cingulum areas in order to aid in straight line access and discovery of the lingual canal. (Illustration by Mr. Oran Suta.)

There are three circumstances in which to consider the use of a labial surface access preparation in the smaller incisors: overdenture abutment, traumatic horizontal fracture of the crown, and planned full coverage restoration after endodontic treatment. This labial approach offers a true straight-line access to the apical region of the canal(s) while maximizing the amount of remaining coronal dentin.

C. When looking for a second canal on a mandibular incisor, the first step is to prepare the access opening as described above. The Endo-Z® bur (Dentsply Sirona, Ballaigues, Switzerland) can be used to extend into the cingulum area for proper lingual access to the site where the second canal would be located. An important adjunct is the use of the operating microscope or loupes with high magnification and illumination to search for the lingual canal on these incisor teeth. The value of higher magnification in these delicate procedures cannot be overstated. The use of the microscope has been found to be instrumental in uncovering 93% of second canals in single-rooted teeth (Rahimi et al. 2013). If troughing is required, an ultrasonic tip is useful to remove tooth structure without impairing operator vision. A sharp endo explorer is very useful in initiating the penetration at the orifice. A size #10 hand file can then be advanced to map out the canal.

D. When faced with a diagnosis of apical periodontitis involving a seemingly intact mandibular incisor, one must consider either trauma, incisal wear (attrition) into the calcified former pulp space, or external cervical invasive resorption (ECIR) as being the cause of the pulp necrosis. Without one of these extraneous insults to the pulp tissue, it is imperative to utilize pulp testing to verify the odontogenic relationship to the lesion. Both cold testing and electric pulp testing (EPT) should be used to confirm the diagnosis of apical periodontitis secondary to pulp necrosis. If a tooth with apical periodontitis responds positively to pulp vitality testing, it is likely that the apical lesion is non-odontogenic in origin. The differential diagnosis of apical periodontitis associated with vital mandibular incisors includes: fibrous dysplasia, cemento-osseous dysplasia, central giant cell granuloma (CGCG), and less frequently, metastatic neoplasms such as multiple myeloma, squamous cell carcinoma, breast cancer, etc. (Özgür et al. 2014). The salient point is to always use a pulp test for any case when an apical periodontitis exists. This is especially true when there is no obvious etiology for the radiographic pathology associated with the tooth. A biopsy of any suspect lesions without odontogenic etiology is highly recommended.

E. The restoration of mandibular central and lateral incisors bears its own set of unique issues. A retrospective study determined that coronal coverage crowns did not significantly improve the success of endodontically treated anterior teeth (Sorensen & Martinoff 1984). Many dentists prefer not to use full coverage on these teeth as there is little coronal dentin to work with after endodontic treatment, and full crown preparation with an aesthetic result in shape and contour is difficult to achieve given the limited space for the restoration. Post and core restorations have been implicated in a higher percentage of root fracture in these small teeth. In fact, mandibular incisors with intact natural crowns exhibit greater resistance to transverse loads compared to teeth with posts and cores (Gluskin et al. 1995). If a post is determined to be necessary due to lack of remaining coronal tooth structure, the narrow mesio-distal width of the central and lateral incisors should limit the ultimate width of the canal or post preparation. Keeping in mind the conservative restoration of a mandibular incisor, the access preparation should preserve mesial and distal coronal dentin, yet the incisal–lingual extension of the preparation must be sufficient for second canal location and straight-line access to the apical root canal. For many reasons the access preparation is the key to long term successful treatment on these diminutive teeth.

References

Çalişkan, M., Pehlivan, Y., Sepetçioğlu, F. et al. (1995) Root canal morphology of human permanent teeth in a Turkish population. *Journal of Endodontics* **21**, 200–204.

Gluskin, A. H., Radke, R. A., Frost, S. L. et al. (1995) The mandibular incisor: Rethinking guidelines for post and core design. *Journal of Endodontics* **21**, 33–37.

Lin, Z., Hu, Q., Wang, T. et al. (2014) Use of CBCT to investigate the root canal morphology of mandibular incisors. *Surgical and Radiologic Anatomy* **36**, 877–882.

Logani, A., Singh, A., Singla, M. et al. (2009) Labial access opening in mandibular teeth – an alternative approach to success. *Quintessence International* **40**, 597–602.

Mahajan, P., Grover, R., Bhandari, S. K. et al. (2016) Management of mandibular lateral incisor with two roots: A case report. *International Journal of Medical and Dental Sciences* **5**, 1093–1097.

Nielsen, C. J. & Shahmohammadi, K. (2005) Effect of mesio-distal chamber dimension on access preparation in mandibular incisors. *Journal of Endodontics* **31**, 88–90.

Özgür, A., Kara, E., Arpaci, R. et al. (2014) Nonodontogenic mandibular lesions: Differentiation based on CT attenuation. *Diagnostic and Interventional Radiology* **20**, 475–480.

Paes da Silva Ramos Fernandes, L. M., Rice, D., Ordinola-Zapata, R. et al. (2014) Detection of various anatomic patterns of root canals in mandibular incisors using digital periapical radiography, 3 cone-beam computed tomographic scanners, and micro-computer tomographic imaging. *Journal of Endodontics* **40**, 42–45.

Rahimi, S., Milani, A. S., Shahi, S. et al. (2013) Prevalence of two root canals in human mandibular anterior teeth in an Iranian population. *Indian Journal of Dental Research* **24**, 234–236.

Shaikh, M. A., Kalhoro, F. A. & Sangi, L. (2014) Frequency of second canal in mandibular lateral incisors (In-vitro). *Pakistan Oral & Dental Journal* **34**, 147–149.

Sorensen, J. A. & Martinoff, J. T. (1984) Intracoronal reinforcement and coronal coverage: A study of endodontically treated teeth. *Journal of Prosthetic Dentistry* **51**, 780–784.

Vertucci, F. J. (1984) Root canal anatomy of the human permanent teeth. *Oral Surgery, Oral Medicine, Oral Pathology, Oral Radiology, and Endodontology* **58**, 589.

9

Non-surgical Root Canal Treatment Case III: Maxillary Anterior/Difficult case (Calcified Coronal ½ Canal System)

Andrew L. Shur

LEARNING OBJECTIVES

- To identify certain preoperative complicating factors that may negatively affect the final outcome as well as long-term success.
- To understand techniques for locating deep calcified canals within a root system.
- To understand how internal bleaching can positively affect aesthetic outcome and the factors affecting its stability.

	Molars			Premolars		Canine	Incisors				Canine	Premolars		Molars		
							Maxillary arch									
Universal tooth designation system	1	2	3	4	5	6	7	8	9	10	11	12	13	14	15	16
International standards organization designation system	18	17	16	15	14	13	12	11	21	22	23	24	25	26	27	28
Palmer method	8⌋	7⌋	6⌋	5⌋	4⌋	3⌋	2⌋	1⌋	⌊1	⌊2	⌊3	⌊4	⌊5	⌊6	⌊7	⌊8
Palmer method	8⌉	7⌉	6⌉	5⌉	4⌉	3⌉	2⌉	1⌉	⌈1	⌈2	⌈3	⌈4	⌈5	⌈6	⌈7	⌈8
International standards organization designation system	48	47	46	45	44	43	42	41	31	32	33	34	35	36	37	38
Universal tooth designation system	32	31	30	29	28	27	26	25	24	23	22	21	20	19	18	17
							Mandibular arch									
		Right								**Left**						

Clinical Cases in Endodontics, First Edition. Edited by Takashi Komabayashi.
© 2018 John Wiley & Sons, Inc. Published 2018 by John Wiley & Sons, Inc.

Chief Complaint

"I would like to lighten the shade of my tooth so it matches with the rest of my teeth."

Medical History

The patient (Pt) was a 58-year-old Caucasian female. Vital signs were as follows: blood pressure (BP) 120/78 mmHg with a pulse of 60 beats per minute (BPM). The Pt was at the time under medical/psychiatric care for mild depression. She reported an allergy to codeine. She was taking the following medications: Celexa®, Lunesta™, Wellbutrin SR®, calcium, vitamin D, and Synthroid®.

The Pt was considered American Society of Anesthesiologists Physical Status Scale (ASA) Class II.

Dental History

The Pt does not recall any history (Hx) of traumatic events affecting tooth #11 and denies previous orthodontic therapy in the recent years. She denies any discomfort associated with the tooth; however, she has noticed the crown of tooth #11 becoming progressively darker over time. The Pt consulted her general dentist who subsequently made the referral for an evaluation for possible endodontic therapy and internal bleaching of tooth #11.

Clinical Evaluation (Diagnostic Procedures)
Examinations
Extra-oral Examination (EOE)

The EOE revealed no abnormal findings.

Intra-oral Examination (IOE)

The perioral and IOE did not yield any abnormal findings. All tissue appeared satisfactory in color and texture. There was no gingival recession present. Periodontal probings measured between 1–3 mm circumferentially around tooth #11. There were no caries, cracks, restorations, or resorptive defects associated with tooth #11. The crown of tooth #11 was much darker than the adjacent teeth as well as the contralateral canine tooth (Figure 9.6).

Diagnostic Tests

Tooth	#10	#11	#12
Percussion	WNL	WNL	WNL
Palpation	WNL	WNL	WNL
Cold	WNL	No response	WNL
Mobility	1	1	1
Bite	–	–	–

WNL: Within normal limits; –: No pain upon biting

Radiographic Findings

Tooth #11 was an unrestored tooth with an intact crown. The bone height appeared WNL, as well as the width of the periodontal ligament (PDL). There were no lateral or apical radiographic findings associated with tooth #11. The canal appeared calcified in the coronal half of the crown and root.

Pretreatment Diagnosis
Pulpal

Pulp Necrosis, tooth #11
(Diagnosis is purely based on a "no cold" response to thermal testing; however, this is to be expected due to the amount of coronal canal calcification)

Apical

Normal Apical Tissue, tooth #11

Treatment Plan
Recommended

Refer Pt back to general dentist for external bleaching and/or possible veneer. Based on the radiographic, clinical, and cone beam-computed tomography (CBCT) examination, no endodontic therapy was recommended at that time.

Alternative

Endodontic therapy on tooth #11 and internal bleaching

Restorative

Veneer or palatal and incisal resin access restoration if endodontic therapy was to be initiated.

Prognosis

Favorable	Questionable	Unfavorable
X		

Clinical Procedures: Treatment Record

First visit (Day 1): A periapical (PA) film was taken of tooth #11 (Figure 9.1). EOE and IOE were performed. The radiographic and clinical examinations yielded no abnormal findings. Since the Pt was asymptomatic and Pt's only issue was the discoloration, no endodontic therapy was recommended. It was recommended that she return to her general dentist for potential external bleaching with the consideration of a cosmetic veneer for the crown discoloration. The Pt understood the recommended treatment (Tx) and planned to consult

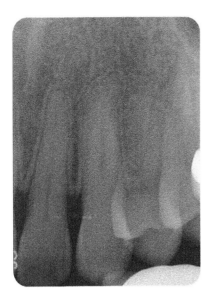

Figure 9.1 Preoperative radiograph: First visit (Day 1).

with her general dentist regarding external bleaching and cosmetic restorative options.

Second visit (2 years, Day 1): The Pt re-presented two years later. Pt was still asymptomatic and a new PA film showed a similar calcified coronal half canal system as previously noted (Figure 9.2). A limited field of view CBCT, Veraviewepocs® 3De, (J. Morita, Kyoto, Japan), was taken which confirmed coronal half canal calcification in the coronal, axial, and sagittal planes (Figures 9.3, 9.4, and 9.5). She reported she consulted with her general dentist regarding the external bleaching and cosmetic options. The general dentist recommended internal bleaching due to the deep discoloration present within the crown. The general

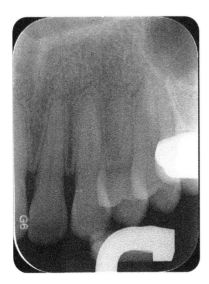

Figure 9.2 Preoperative radiograph: Second visit (2 years, Day 1).

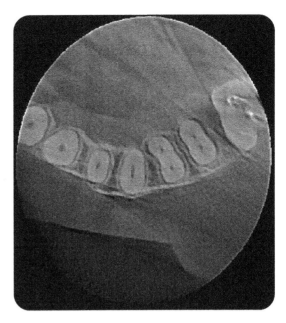

Figure 9.3 Axial CBCT slice mid-root through canal tooth #11.

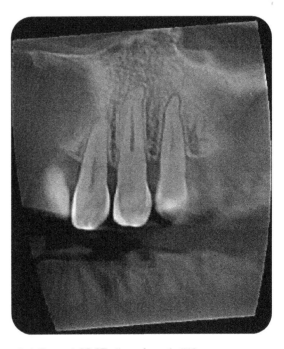

Figure 9.4 Frontal CBCT slice of tooth #11.

dentist did not feel she could obtain an adequate aesthetic result with external bleaching, and was hesitant to prepare an intact crown for a cosmetic veneer. The potential risks of endodontic therapy on tooth #11 due to the calcified coronal 1/2 canal system were explained to the Pt. She was made aware that perforation was a potential risk; however, I explained that I would not become overly aggressive searching for the calcified canal since she was asymptomatic and the radiographic and CBCT examination appeared WNL.

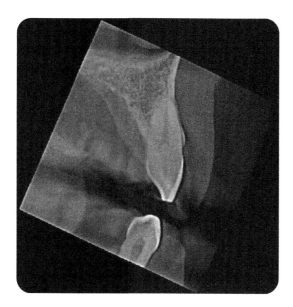

Figure 9.5 Sagittal CBCT slice of tooth #11.

The Pt signed consent for endodontic therapy and internal bleaching, and Tx was scheduled.

Third visit (Day 26): The Pt presented for Tx. BP and pulse were taken and recorded. Anesthesia was achieved with 2 x 1.8 cc lidocaine (lido) and 1:100,000 epinephrine (epi) administered via local infiltration. Tooth #11 was isolated with a rubber dam (RD). A surgical operating microscope was utilized and a palatal endodontic access towards the incisal was prepared in tooth #11. Clinically, the canal system was calcified in the crown and coronal root structure, as evidenced from the radiographic and CBCT examination. Using long shank small burs, Ethylenediaminetetraacetic acid (EDTA), sodium hypochlorite (NaOCl), and the surgical operating microscope (SOM), I was able to discern the calcified pulp canal space as a dark ring of dentin centrally placed within the root. Carefully following the dark dentin with the long shank burs and ultrasonic instruments, the pulp canal was eventually located. No excess dentin appeared to be removed from the mid root or peri-cervical region of the tooth, and the root was not perforated in the process. The pulp tissue in the root appeared necrotic as it was not the typical pink healthy tissue in a "normal tooth." The root canal system was shaped with a combination of rotary instruments and stainless steel hand files. The canal was irrigated with 5.25% NaOCl and 17% EDTA. The irritants were activated and the canal was dried with micro-suction and paper points. Patency was checked with a size #8 hand file. The canal was obturated with vertical

compaction of warm gutta-percha (GP) with AH Plus® Root Canal Sealer (Dentsply Sirona, Konstanz, Germany) to within a few millimeters of the cementoenamel junction (CEJ). Cavit™ (3M, Two Harbors, MN, USA) was placed over the GP up to the CEJ to act as a barrier for the bleach. It was, and remains, the opinion of the clinician that Cavit™ appears to serve as well as glass ionomer or resin as a protective orifice seal for the purpose of internal bleaching. Sodium perborate and superoxyl were mixed and carefully placed within the access cavity. The access was sealed with Cavit™ as a temporary restoration. All postoperative instructions were reviewed and the Pt was booked in for a "bleach check" appointment.

Fourth visit (1-week follow-up): The Pt presented for a bleach check. The tooth was asymptomatic. Although the color had improved since the initial visit (Figures 9.6, 9.7 and 9.8), the crown was still darker and the Pt desired to continue bleaching. Tooth #11 was re-isolated with a RD. No anesthesia was administered. The Cavit™ was removed and the access cavity was irrigated with sterile water. A fresh mixture of sodium perborate and

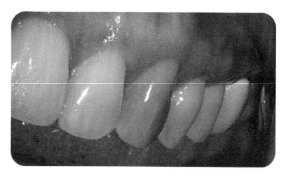

Figure 9.6 Clinical photograph showing discoloration of tooth #11 due to internal calcification.

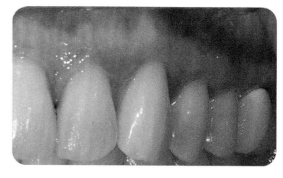

Figure 9.7 Clinical photograph showing tooth #11 after completion of internal bleaching.

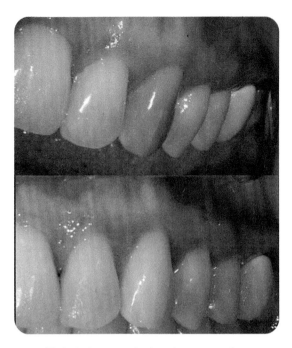

Figure 9.8 Clinical photograph showing comparison pre- and post-internal bleaching of tooth #11. (Top: pre-internal bleaching, Bottom: post-internal bleaching)

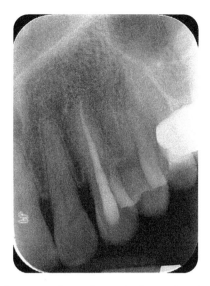

Figure 9.9 Postoperative radiograph of completed endodontic therapy of tooth #11.

Post-Treatment Evaluation

A one-year recall PA radiograph was e-mailed from the referring dentist for review (Figure 9.10). The Pt was not seen in the office for a recall examination at that time.

Seventh visit (4-year follow-up): The Pt presented for a recall examination four years after the Tx was complete. She was asymptomatic and the PA radiograph of tooth #11 appeared WNL (Figure 9.11). The surrounding periodontal tissues also appeared WNL. The color of tooth #11 had remained stable within the four-year period (Figure 9.12). The Pt was placed on another one-year recall.

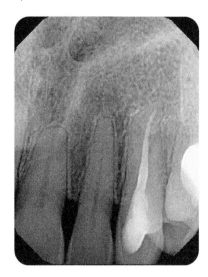

Figure 9.10 One-year recall radiograph emailed from a referring dentist.

superoxyl was placed into the access and sealed with Cavit™. The Pt scheduled for another "bleach check" appointment.

Fifth visit (2-week follow-up): The Pt presented for another bleach check. The tooth was still asymptomatic. Although the color had improved since the first bleach application, the crown was still slightly darker and the Pt desired to continue bleaching. Tooth #11 was re-isolated with a RD. No anesthesia was administered. The Cavit™ was removed and the access cavity was irrigated with sterile water. A fresh mixture of sodium perborate and superoxyl was placed into the access and sealed with Cavit™. The Pt scheduled for another "bleach check" appointment.

Sixth visit (4-week follow-up): The Pt presented and was happy with the color of tooth #11. The tooth was re-isolated with a RD. No anesthesia was administered. The Cavit™ was removed and the access was flushed with sterile water. The access was restored with bonded composite resin and contoured smooth. The occlusion was checked and adjusted as necessary. A postoperative PA radiograph was taken (Figure 9.9). The Pt was placed on a standard recall.

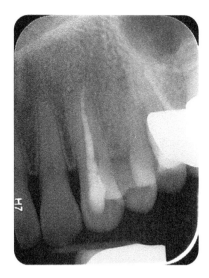

Figure 9.11 Four-year recall radiograph, tooth #11.

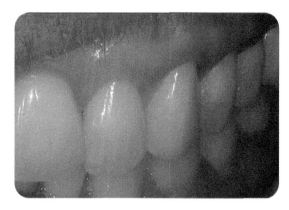

Figure 9.12 Four-year recall clinical photograph, tooth #11.

Self-Study Questions

A. How does a surgical operating microscope (SOM) help the clinician locate calcified canals within a root?

B. How can a CBCT scan help guide a clinician to locate deep calcified canals within a root?

C. What are some indications for internal bleaching?

D. Why is it important to recall endodontic cases after more than six months to one year?

E. Explain why pulp canal obliteration (PCO) can be a challenge for the clinician treating a given tooth, and list some tools and instruments that may help make treatment possible.

Answers to Self-Study Questions

A. The SOM provides the clinician with superior illumination and magnification when compared to dental loupes, an overhead light source, or the naked eye. Calcified canals can easily be addressed by utilizing the SOM (Carr & Murgel 2010). Astute clinicians can learn visual skills required to discern dentin from calcified pulp, relying on dentinal color changes, translucency, and refractive properties to help locate remnants of calcified pulpal tissue. Previously, perforations or over-enlargement of accesses have resulted in decreasing the lifespan of a calcified tooth; however, the SOM makes these types of cases routine and more predictable.

B. A PA radiograph shows structures in 2-D, whereas a CBCT shows structures in 3-D. When carefully drilling down a root to locate a deep canal, a 2-D radiograph will help guide the clinician in a mesial to distal direction only. Although this information is helpful, it tells the clinician nothing about the buccal–palatal orientation. Although the clinician may think he or she is nearing the canal on a PA radiographic, the clinician may in fact be close to perforating the root, usually towards the buccal. Also, CBCT software frequently has "measuring tools" to help estimate distances from the incisal edge reference point to the deep canal orifice. A sagittal or axial slice taken during the procedure can often help guide the clinician safely towards the deep canal within the confines of the root (Nallapati 2015).

C. Despite some historically bad press in the literature, if done properly, internal bleaching can be a safe and effective procedure for improving the aesthetic outcome of a darkened anterior tooth. Use of unheated bleach is recommended, as well as the use of a protective barrier a few millimeters thick of restorative material at the CEJ level within the tooth and root. Indications for internal bleaching can include intrinsic staining from blood breakdown products, restorative materials, excessive fluoride,

certain medications, and pulp canal obliteration post trauma (Abbott & Heah 2009). Various types of staining respond well to internal bleaching and can remain stable for years.

D. Historically, recall rates in endodontic private practices tend to be low. Most endodontists tend to recall cases at six months, and possibly one year, if they recall patients at all. However, the clinician should make every effort to obtain "long-term" recalls. This case displays a four-year recall at the time of publication, and although not quite "long term," it can be considered "intermediate term." A six-month or one-year recall can help the clinician evaluate apical healing on a given case (Orstavik 1996); however, endodontists should be concerned about tooth survivability after endodontics. A short-term recall will help the clinician discern whether a case may be successfully working from a process-centered point of view; however, a long-term recall is required for properly assessing the outcomes from a patient-centered perspective.

E. PCO presents a challenge to treatment on several levels (McCabe & Dummer 2012). Roughly 4–24% of teeth can display some form of PCO post trauma. It may be difficult to rely on sensibility testing with teeth that have undergone PCO, and technically, these teeth may be difficult to treat as locating the actual canal can often be challenging. From a treatment planning angle, knowing when to treat may also pose a challenge to the clinician, i.e., treat at the first sign of PCO although the tooth is completely asymptomatic? It is recommended that treatment for teeth with PCO only be initiated if there are clinical signs and symptoms indicative of a periapical disease. Tools and instruments that may aid the clinician in successfully treating cases with PCO can include (but are not limited to): SOM, CBCT, long shank small burs, EDTA, ultrasonics, and small diameter (size #6 and size #8) stiff hand files.

References

Abbott, P. & Heah, S. Y. (2009) Internal bleaching of teeth: an analysis of 255 teeth. *Australian Dental Journal* **54**, 326–333.

Carr, G. B. & Murgel, C. A. (2010) The use of the operating microscope in endodontics. *Dental Clinics of North America* **54**, 191–214.

McCabe, P. S. & Dummer, P. M. (2012) Pulp canal obliteration: An endodontic diagnosis and treatment challenge. *International Endodontic Journal* **45**, 177–197.

Nallapati, S. (2015) Clinical management of calcified teeth. In: *Best Practices in Endodontics: A Desk Reference* (eds. R. S. Schwartz & V. Canakapalli), pp. 124–128. Chicago: Quintessence.

Orstavik, D. (1996) Time-course and risk analysis of the development and healing of chronic apical periodontitis in man. *International Endodontic Journal* **29**, 150–155.

10

Non-surgical Root Canal Treatment Case IV: Maxillary Premolar

Daniel Chavarría-Bolaños, David Masuoka-Ito, and Amaury J. Pozos-Guillén

LEARNING OBJECTIVES
- To understand a clinical and pharmacological approach to the non-surgical root canal treatment of maxillary premolars.
- To understand the essential aspects of endodontic diagnosis of maxillary premolars.
- To understand aspects of preclinical preparation for non-surgical root canal treatment (NSRCT) of maxillary premolars, including anatomical considerations and clinical and pharmacological approaches.
- To analyze different considerations for the selection of local anesthesia techniques based on the best available evidence.
- To understand the clinical management of NSRCT, including mechanical preparation, irrigation, and obturation techniques.
- To understand restorative and functional aspects that will affect the behavior and prognosis of maxillary premolars that have undergone non-surgical root canal treatment.

	Molars			Premolars		Canine	Incisors				Canine	Premolars		Molars		
							Maxillary arch									
Universal tooth designation system	1	2	3	4	5	6	7	8	9	10	11	12	13	14	15	16
International standards organization designation system	18	17	16	15	14	13	12	11	21	22	23	24	25	26	27	28
Palmer method	8	7	6	5	4	3	2	1	1	2	3	4	5	6	7	8
Palmer method	8	7	6	5	4	3	2	1	1	2	3	4	5	6	7	8
International standards organization designation system	48	47	46	45	44	43	42	41	31	32	33	34	35	36	37	38
Universal tooth designation system	32	31	30	29	28	27	26	25	24	23	22	21	20	19	18	17
							Mandibular arch									
	Right										**Left**					

Clinical Cases in Endodontics, First Edition. Edited by Takashi Komabayashi.
© 2018 John Wiley & Sons, Inc. Published 2018 by John Wiley & Sons, Inc.

Chief Complaint

"I feel a sharp pain in this area (pointing to the area below the zygomatic bone, at the level of tooth #5). It hurts all day especially when I bite with that tooth (pointing to tooth #5). I took a couple of analgesics but they failed to control it. This has been my nightmare for the last week."

Medical History

The patient (Pt) was a 38-year old male. He did not report any substantial medical condition.

The Pt was considered American Society of Anesthesiologists Physical Status Scale (ASA) Class I.

Dental History

Pt presented with multiple dental treatments throughout the oral cavity. Specifically, tooth #5 presented a mesio-occluso-distal (MOD) amalgam restoration that was placed several years before. (The Pt did not know the exact date).

Clinical Evaluation (Diagnostic Procedures)
Examinations
Extra-oral Examination (EOE)

EOE revealed no cervical lymphadenopathy. There was no tenderness of masticatory muscles upon palpation. Perioral/intraoral soft tissue showed no signs of inflammation, pigmentation, or any other identifiable abnormalities. Extra-oral soft tissues were healthy and asymptomatic. Temporomandibular joint (TMJ) exhibited no pain, sounds, or deviation upon maximum opening.

Intraoral examination (IOE)

IOE exhibited no gingival inflammation around the right maxillary 1st premolar (tooth #5), but erythematosus aspect was observed. Periodontal depth of 2 mm was seen all over the teeth cervical contour after probing. The Pt's hygiene was acceptable. Physiologic mobility was observed.

Diagnostic Tests

Tooth	#5	#4 (control)	#12 (control)
Percussion	Tenderness	Normal	Normal
Palpation	Normal	Normal	Normal
Cold	No response	Normal	Normal

Teeth #3 and #6 were not tested since they were asymptomatic and presented endodontic treatment.

Radiographic Findings

Radiographically it was possible to observe root canal treatments (RCT) in teeth #3 and #6. Tooth #4 showed normal vitality, and a well-adjusted amalgam restoration. No teeth in the upper right (UR) quadrant showed the presence of caries.

Tooth #5 showed the presence of an MOD amalgam restoration (Figure 10.1), also widened apical periodontal ligament. No carious lesions were identified beneath the amalgam restoration.

Pretreatment Diagnosis
Pulpal

Pulp Necrosis, tooth #5

Apical

Symptomatic Apical Periodontitis, tooth #5

Treatment Plan
Recommended

Emergency: None
Definitive: Non-surgical Root Canal Therapy (NSRCT) of tooth #5

Alternative

Extraction

Restorative

Composite restoration

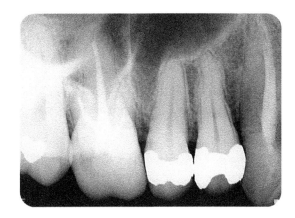

Figure 10.1 Initial radiograph. Tooth #5 showed the presence of a mesio-occlusal-distal (MOD) amalgam restoration. No carious lesions are observed under the restoration. Widened apical periodontal ligament is observed.

Prognosis

Favorable	Questionable	Unfavorable
X		

Tooth structure was well maintained, the occlusion was atraumatic, and no chronic apical lesion was observed.

Clinical Procedures: Treatment Record

First visit (Day 1): Before any clinical intervention, a full medical history was obtained, and the informed consent was signed by the Pt. A brief explanation of all procedures was given to the Pt. It was decided to use a preemptive analgesia protocol, by asking the Pt to take 25 mg of dexketoprofen trometamol (Stein Corp., Cartago, Costa Rica) before the treatment. After 15 minutes, local anesthesia was administered by infiltration of one cartridge of mepivacaine hydrochloride 2% with adrenaline (epinephrine) 1:100,000 (Septodont, Lancaster, PA, USA). After five minutes, the tooth was evaluated to assure that the anesthetic effect was achieved by repeating the percussion test. Complete isolation was performed by using a latex rubber dam and clamp #2 (Hu-Friedy, Chicago, IL, USA).

The existing amalgam was removed using a #6 carbide round bur. The remaining tooth structure was evaluated for the presence of fissures and fractures using a surgical microscope. Any residual caries were removed, and further isolation was achieved using OpalDam® (Ultradent, South Jordan, UT, USA) light-cured flowable dental dam material. Immediately, the endodontic access was performed by using a cylindrical diamond bur, in conjunction with copious irrigation of 3.5% sodium hypochlorite (NaOCl) solution. The pulp chamber was rinsed, and two root canals (buccal and palatal) were identified and located using ultrasonic diamond instruments. Both canals were gently rinsed with 3.5% NaOCl before any instrumentation.

Once the initial disinfection was completed, the working lengths (WL) of both root canals were determined by using an electronic apex locator Root ZX® II (J. Morita, Kyoto, Japan). A size #10 hand file coupled to the electronic apex locator was gently introduced into each canal until the device indicated the locations of the apical constrictions. WLs were determined as 22 mm and 21 mm for buccal and palatal root canals respectively. Manual instrumentation of the root canals was performed, beginning with a size #15 file and finishing with a size #25 file. Between each file, copious irrigation with 3.5% NaOCl was done, and patency was established with a size #10 file. After

manual instrumentation, rotary preparation was done with the full sequence of ProTaper® Universal (Dentsply Sirona, Ballaigues, Switzerland), until the apical portion was instrumented to an F2 file. As with manual files, between each instrument, copious irrigation was used and patency was confirmed. Just after the final preparation was done with an F2 file, passive ultrasonic irrigation was used. For this procedure, a stainless steel non-diamond ultrasonic tip (Satelec, Merignac, France) was adjusted 3 mm coronal to the working length. Both root canals were filled with NaOCl and passive ultrasonic activation was performed for 30 seconds (avoiding the contact of the instrument with dentin walls). Once the root canals were irrigated and prepared, a final irrigation with 17% Ethylenediaminetetraacetic acid (EDTA) was used, leaving the irrigant for 30 seconds. Finally, the canals were rinsed with NaOCl. The root canals were then dried by using aspiration with Capillary™ tips (Ultradent, South Jordan, UT, USA) and ProTaper® Universal F2 paper points (Dentsply Sirona, Ballaigues, Switzerland).

For the obturation phase, continuous wave technique was selected by using a B & L Biotech obturation device (B & L, McKinney, TX, USA). Two F2 gutta-percha (GP) points were adjusted. GP points were coated with a thin layer of root canal sealer TopSeal® (Dentsply Sirona, Konstanz, Germany) and were placed into the root canal. The apical third of each canal was obturated with the Alpha unit (B & L, McKinney, TX, USA), followed by gentle vertical compaction with #5 and #7 Schilder® pluggers (Obtura Spartan Endodontics, Algonquin, IL, USA). The remaining canal was obturated using warm GP with the Beta unit (B & L, McKinney, TX, USA), followed by vertical compaction. A radiograph was taken to confirm appropriate obturation of the root canal (Figure 10.2).

After obturation, the remaining sealer was cleaned, and a dry sterile cotton pellet was placed in the pulp chamber. Cavit™ temporary restorative material (3M, North Rhine-Westphalia, Germany) was then placed in the endodontic access and the Pt was then instructed not to eat or drink for 2 hours following treatment, and to visit the clinician as soon as possible for the permanent restoration. A final radiograph was taken (Figure 10.3).

Since the Pt reported preoperatory pain, a pharmacologic analgesic protocol of multiple doses was selected by using an analgesic combination (multimodal approach). The Pt was asked to take 25 mg of dexketoprofen trometamol (Laboratorios Stein, Cartago,

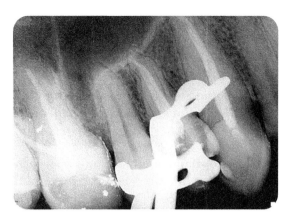

Figure 10.2 Radiographic evaluation of the obturation. Immediately after the injection and compaction of warm gutta-percha, a periapical radiograph was taken to confirm the obturation of the case. Some sealer extruded from the root canal can be observed in the apical region.

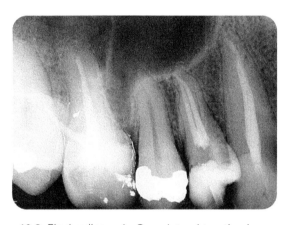

Figure 10.3 Final radiograph. Complete obturation is observed. Coronally, one can observe the space where the sterile cotton pellet was placed and the temporary restoration.

Costa Rica), combined with 500 mg of paracetamol (Laboratorios Stein, Cartago, Costa Rica) every eight hours for the next three days. The Pt was advised to continue taking dexketoprofen for an additional two days if pain and discomfort persisted. The Pt was advised to return for evaluation if symptoms persisted beyond this five-day period.

After one week, the clinician overseeing the final restoration was contacted to ask about the improvement of the Pt. The clinician reported that the Pt was asymptomatic and had taken the prescribed medication for only the first 3 days. Tooth #5 had been successfully restored using composite restorative material A2 Filtek™ Z350 (3M, Two Harbors, MN, USA).

Working length, apical size, and obturation technique

Canal	Working Length	Apical Size, Taper	Obturation Materials and Techniques
B	22.0 mm	ProTaper® Universal F2	TopSeal® sealer, Vertical compaction
P	21.0 mm	ProTaper® Universal F2	TopSeal® sealer, Vertical compaction

Post-Treatment Evaluation

Second visit (29-month follow-up): The Pt returned for a control appointment. Clinical examination revealed a normal healthy periodontium and the absence of caries in teeth #4, #5, and #6. Tooth #5 was asymptomatic, and palpation and percussion tests were normal. The composite restoration on tooth #5 was adjusted and functional. Radiographically, the periapical tissues did not show any sign of inflammation or pathologic changes (Figure 10.4).

Third visit (63-month follow-up): The Pt returned for reevaluation. There were no adverse changes in the clinical and radiographic evaluation of the tooth since the first visit (Figure 10.5). The Pt was scheduled to reappoint after a period of one year, for continued evaluation.

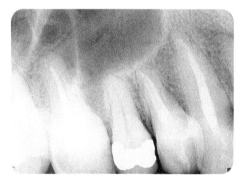

Figure 10.4 Twenty-nine-month follow-up. Tooth #5 showed a positive prognosis after the root canal treatment. The restoration was well-adapted and the extruded sealer had resorbed.

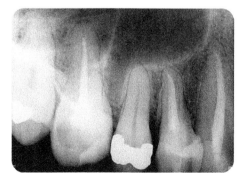

Figure 10.5 Sixty-three-month follow-up. Tooth #5 did not show any sign of pathological process related to the root canal treatment. The tooth is still asymptomatic, with normal occlusal function.

Self-Study Questions

A. List different non-odontogenic reasons that must be considered in the differential diagnosis of maxillary premolar pain.

B. Summarize important anatomical features that may be expected in root canal treatment of maxillary premolars.

C. List some considerations governing the selection of the anesthetic solution for the endodontic treatment of maxillary premolars.

D. What advantages does the use of pre-emptive analgesia offer for the endodontic management of painful teeth?

E. What is the optimal pharmacologic approach for the post-operative management of symptomatic endodontic pathologies?

Answers to Self-Study Questions

A. Although most dental pain is related to endodontic and/or periodontal conditions, it is mandatory that the clinician consider and rule out other non-odontogenic causes that can present as dental pain. According to Okeson (2014), some common non-odontogenic pains are:

- Localized myofascial toothache (especially in maxillary posterior teeth when the masseter and temporal muscles are involved).
- Non-odontogenic sinusitis (caused by inflammation of the ostium and thus compression of nociceptors causing maxillary teeth pain).
- Migraine (specially midface migraine, which may cause direct pain over maxillary teeth).
- Neuropathic pain (episodic conditions such as trigeminal neuralgia or continuous localized pathologies like atypical odontalgia).
- Psychogenic pain (where no tissue lesion is present, but the patient replicates psychological problems as tooth pain).

B. Maxillary premolars may exhibit different anatomies that can transform a radiographically "simple" case into a "hard one." To predict the real anatomy is almost impossible based only on the clinical and radiographic examinations. Even to compare the anatomy of these teeth within different populations is difficult. A recent review (Ahmad & Alenezi 2016) summarizes important aspects of the anatomy of maxillary premolars. Most of the maxillary 1st premolars have one (41.7%) or two (56.6%) roots; however, the number of root canals is not related to the number of roots: 86.6% of maxillary 1st premolars have two root canals, for example. Clinically, it is important to remember that the most common anatomic variation is the presence of a third root. Apically speaking, the majority of the teeth had either one foramen (29.5%) or two foramina (68.6%), and the majority of these foramina (66.6%) did not coincide with the apical root tip (Ahmad & Alenezi 2016).

C. A successful anesthetic blockade before endodontic treatment is crucial, and the most important aspect is anesthetic selection (Malamed 2013). When possible, the use of vasoconstrictors is always recommended in order to increase the duration of the effect and reduce the toxicity of anesthesia. In cases of local inflammation (due to pulpal necrosis or pulpitis) where the pH is low, choosing a molecule with low pKa is beneficial. In this sense, mepivacaine offers important advantages for the blockade of previously inflamed maxillary premolars. With a lower vasodilatory effect, a low pKa, and high lipophilicity, this anesthetic represents an important option.

D. Pre-emptive analgesia offers important advantages for the management of painful endodontic cases. The first indication for this treatment is the presence of preoperatory pain, a condition related to anesthetic failure (Hargreaves & Keiser 2002) and intraoperative / postoperative pain (Pak & White 2011). Preadministration of several non-steroidal anti-inflammatory drugs (NSAIDs) such as ibuprofen demonstrate an increase in the anesthetic blockade (Noguera-Gonzalez et al. 2013). Pre-emptive analgesia also prolongs the blockade duration, improving the post-operative period for the patient. Another important advantage is the decrease in post-operative pharmacological treatment, thus diminishing possible side effects (Sagiroglu 2011).

E. In cases of moderate to severe preoperatory acute pain, when the anesthetic blockade was not fully obtained, when the clinical procedure was painful, or when mishaps happen, postoperative pharmacological treatment is advisable. Such an approach must combine not only the right molecules, but also the optimal protocols in order to successfully control the pain.

The use of NSAIDs is still the first option to manage pain (Laskarides 2016). The molecules of several substances, such as ibuprofen, ketorolac, dexketprofen trometamol, and etoricoxib, among others, have been analyzed, with similar and acceptable clinical results. However, the final molecule of choice is related to the systemic condition of the patient including consideration of concomitant systemic diseases, history of allergies, and/or other medical treatments of the patient. If the use of NSAIDs is not indicated, the use of paracetamol or dual analgesics like tramadol may be the second choice. If the expected effect is not achieved by using a single-drug approach, it is advisable to consider multimodal strategies, specifically analgesic combinations (Buvanendran & Kroin 2009). If NSAIDs can be used, then combining them with paracetamol or tramadol is recommended. If not, combining tramadol and paracetamol is also recommended; however, this combination lacks anti-inflammatory efficacy.

A "dynamic" approach for the selection of protocols is advisable. A dynamic approach individualizes each treatment depending on the needs of the patient, since there are no standard prescriptions that can be generalized to all patients. For example, if the pre-operatory pain was severe, with a history of poor pharmacological pain response, then the use of multiple doses is advisable to manage the pain expected for the first 48 to 72 hours. In such a case, the protocol could involve analgesic combinations for the first doses. If the patient reported improvement in the short term, then one of the two compounds combined could be eliminated (i.e., continue only with the NSAID until complete absence of symptoms is achieved).

References

Ahmad, I. A. & Alenezi, M. A. (2016) Root and root canal morphology of maxillary first premolars: A literature review and clinical considerations. *Journal of Endodontics* **42**, 861–872.

Buvanendran, A. & Kroin, J. S. (2009) Multimodal analgesia for controlling acute postoperative pain. *Current Opinion in Anaesthesiology* **22**, 588–593.

Hargreaves, K. M. & Keiser, K. (2002) Local anesthetic failure in endodontics. *Endodontic Topics* **1**, 26–39.

Laskarides, C. (2016) Update on analgesic medication for adult and pediatric dental patients. *Dental Clinics of North America* **60**, 347–366.

Malamed, S. (2013) Pharmacology of local anesthetics. In: *Handbook of Local Anesthesia* (ed. S. F. Malamed), 6th edn, pp. 25–38. St. Louis, MO: Mosby Elsevier.

Noguera-Gonzalez, D., Cerda-Cristerna, B. I., Chavarria-Bolanos, D. *et al.* (2013) Efficacy of preoperative ibuprofen on the success of inferior alveolar nerve block in patients with symptomatic irreversible pulpitis: A randomized clinical trial. *International Endodontic Journal* **46**, 1056–1062.

Okeson, J. P. (2014) Dental pains. In: *Bell's Oral and Facial Pain* (ed. J. P. Okeson), 7th edn, pp. 249–285. Chicago: Quintessence.

Pak, J. G. & White, S. N. (2011). Pain prevalence and severity before, during, and after root canal treatment: A systematic review. *Journal of Endodontics* **37**, 429–438.

Sagiroglu, G. (2011) Comparing early postoperative period analgesic effect of dexketoprofene trometamol and lornoxicam in mediastinoscopy cases. *Eurasian Journal of Medicine* **43**, 23–26.

11

Non-surgical Root Canal Treatment Case V: Mandibular Premolar

Takashi Okiji

LEARNING OBJECTIVES

■ To describe the root and root canal morphology of the mandibular premolar.

■ To describe the anatomical relationship between the mandibular premolar and the inferior alveolar nerve.

■ To understand the complications associated with neural damage during root canal treatment of mandibular premolars.

	Molars			Premolars		Canine	Incisors				Canine	Premolars		Molars		
							Maxillary arch									
Universal tooth designation system	1	2	3	4	5	6	7	8	9	10	11	12	13	14	15	16
International standards organization designation system	18	17	16	15	14	13	12	11	21	22	23	24	25	26	27	28
Palmer method	8⌋	7⌋	6⌋	5⌋	4⌋	3⌋	2⌋	1⌋	⌊1	⌊2	⌊3	⌊4	⌊5	⌊6	⌊7	⌊8
Palmer method	8⌉	7⌉	6⌉	5⌉	4⌉	3⌉	2⌉	1⌉	⌈1	⌈2	⌈3	⌈4	⌈5	⌈6	⌈7	⌈8
International standards organization designation system	48	47	46	45	44	43	42	41	31	32	33	34	35	36	37	38
Universal tooth designation system	32	31	30	29	28	27	26	25	24	23	22	21	20	19	18	17
							Mandibular arch									
	Right										**Left**					

Chief Complaint

"My lower right jaw was swollen and painful and I had the affected part operated on by a surgeon. Now the pain and swelling are almost gone, but I still feel numbness in my lower lip."

Medical History

The patient (Pt) was a 71-year-old female. Medical history was not significant, except for hypertension that was controlled with a calcium channel blocker. The Pt had no known drug allergies (NKDA).

The Pt was considered American Society of Anesthesiologists Physical Status Scale (ASA) Class II.

Dental History

Pt had been referred by an oral surgeon for the endodontic treatment of tooth #29. Approximately one month previously, the Pt had been referred to the oral surgeon by a general dentist for the treatment (Tx) of severe spontaneous pain and swelling of the right mandible associated with a loss of sensitivity on the right side of the skin and mucosa of her lower lip. The general dentist made an opening in the pulp chamber, which was left unsealed. The oral surgeon made an incision in the fluctuant swelling under a diagnosis of an acute apical abscess originating in tooth #29, and prescribed a cephem antibiotic (Flomox®). The Pt's swelling and pain disappeared after a few days. However, the numbness was still present 14 days after the first visit and the Pt was given a prescription for vitamin B12 for the management of paresthesia. Then the oral surgeon referred the Pt to the Department of Endodontics for endodontic Tx of tooth #29.

Clinical Evaluation (Diagnostic Procedures)
Examinations
Extra-oral Examination (EOE)

No swelling or lymphadenopathy of the submandibular and neck areas was found. Soft tissue sensitivity, as evaluated with a dental probe, revealed a reduced tactile sensitivity in the skin of the right mental region and lower lip.

Intra-oral Examination (IOE)

Reduction of tactile sensation in the oral mucosa up to the midline was recognized. The oral hygiene of the Pt was poor. Tooth #29 had an unsealed access cavity on its occlusal surface and an old composite filling on its buccal (B) cervical area (Figure 11.1). There were carious lesions on its mesial (M), lingual (L), and distal (D) cervical surfaces close to the gingival margin. The

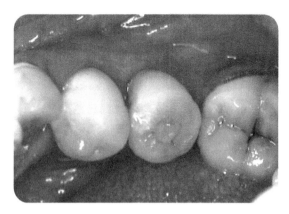

Figure 11.1 Preoperative clinical photograph of tooth #29.

probing pocket depths were 3–4 mm around the circumference of the tooth.

Diagnostic Tests

Tooth	#31	#29	#28
Percussion	–	+	–
Palpation	–	+	–
Cold	+	–	+
EPT	+	–	+

EPT: Electric pulp test; +: Response to percussion or palpation, and normal response to cold and EPT; -: No response to percussion, palpation, cold, or EPT

Radiographic Findings

Periapical (PA) radiograph revealed that tooth #29 had a single root and root canal that was curved at the apical one-fourth to the D at approximately 30° (Figure 11.2). There was a radiolucency approximately 5 mm in diameter at the PA area of tooth #29. At the M cervical region, there was a deep carious lesion showing close proximity to the pulp chamber. The right premolar area on the panoramic radiograph showed distortion, but it was suggested that the periapical radiolucency (PARL) was in close proximity to the mental foramen (Figure 11.3). Computerized tomography (CT) scans demonstrated that the B cortical plate of the apical region of tooth #29 was interrupted, and the PARL involving tooth #29 showed communication with the mandibular canal (Figure 11.4A, B).

Pretreatment Diagnosis
Pulpal

Pulp Necrosis, tooth #29

Apical

Symptomatic Apical Periodontitis, tooth #29 (Associated with Mental Nerve Paresthesia)

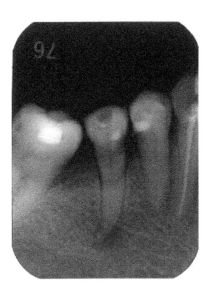

Figure 11.2 Preoperative periapical radiograph of tooth #29.

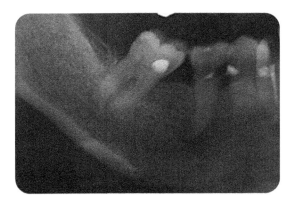

Figure 11.3 Preoperative panoramic radiograph showing mandibular right premolar and molar regions.

Treatment Plan
Recommended

Emergency: No treatment
Definitive: Non-Surgical Endodontic Treatment

Alternative

No treatment

Restorative

Cast metal post and core, and a full metal crown

Prognosis

Favorable	Questionable	Unfavorable
	X	

Since there was a possibility that extraction of tooth #29 would exacerbate the paresthesia of the mental region, and the tooth was deemed to be restorable, non-surgical endodontic Tx was planned to control PA inflammation, with an expectation of subsequent resolution of mental nerve paresthesia.

Clinical Procedures: Treatment Record

First visit (Day 1): The caries of the proximal and L cervical regions was first removed with low-speed round burs and excavators, and the cavities were temporarily sealed with a temporary filling material (Caviton®, GC Corporation, Tokyo, Japan). The tooth was then isolated with a rubber dam (RD). The access cavity was slightly enlarged using a diamond bur with a high-speed handpiece, and the coronal pulp chamber was irrigated

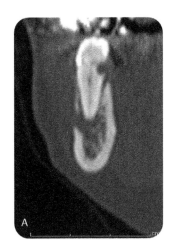
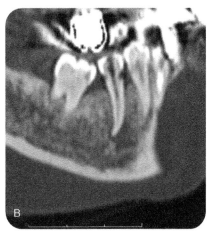

Figure 11.4 Preoperative multi-slice CT images of tooth #29. Coronal view (A) and sagittal view (B). The B cortical plate of the apical region of the tooth #29 is interrupted, and the PARL involving tooth #29 shows communication with the mandibular canal.

with approximately 1.5% sodium hypochlorite (NaOCl) (Neo Cleaner, Neo Dental, Tokyo, Japan), diluted with sterile saline. Approximately, the coronal one-third of the canal was then flared with Gates-Glidden drills (#2 to #4 in a step-back manner), and again irrigated with NaOCl. Instrumentation of the canal was performed by a modified crown-down pressureless technique using stainless steel K-files (Mani, Tochigi, Japan) and nickel titanium (NiTi) rotary instruments (K3™, Sybron, Orange, CA, USA), rotated at 300 rpm using a torque-control motor (TCM Endo, Nouvag, Goldach, Switzerland). The canal was first instrumented with K-files of progressively smaller sizes (#35 to #20). The files were inserted into the canal and rotated passively at the length of resistance. A provisional working length (WL) of approximately 3 mm short of the apex was determined. Then, K3 instruments (size#/ taper) #45/.04, #40/.04, #35/.04, and #30/.04 were used sequentially in a crown-down manner until the #35/.04 instrument reached to the provisional WL. The canal was irrigated with NaOCl at every file change. Following preparation to the provisional WL, passive ultrasonic irrigation was performed to activate NaOCl using an ultrasonic device (ENAC, Osada, Tokyo, Japan) and a size #20 ultrasonic file (Osada, Tokyo, Japan). Final WL was then determined with an electronic apex locator (Root ZX® II, J.Morita, Kyoto, Japan) and a size #10 K-file. Following glide path preparation with a size #15 K-file, the canal was again instrumented with K3 instruments (size/ taper, #35/.04, #30/.04, and #25/.04) in a crown-down manner until the size #25/.04 taper instrument reached the working length. The canal was irrigated with NaOCl after each file change. The root canal was dried with paper points, dressed with calcium hydroxide (Ca(OH)$_2$) paste (Calcipex®, Nippon Shika Yakuhin, Shimonoseki, Japan), and the tooth was provisionally sealed with Caviton®.

Second visit (Day 10): The Tx at the first visit was uneventful, and the paresthetic symptoms were resolving with a slightly reduced sensation of the affected area. The tooth was isolated with an RD, the temporary restoration in the access cavity was removed, and the Ca(OH)$_2$ dressing was removed with K-files and irrigation with a syringe and an ultrasonic device using NaOCl as an irrigant. The canal was then instrumented to a size #35/.04 taper with K3 instruments in a crown-down manner. Subsequently, the root canal was dried with paper points and filled with gutta-percha (GP) points (GC Corporation, Tokyo,

Japan) and a zinc oxide non-eugenol sealer (Canals®-N, Showa Yakuhin Kako, Tokyo, Japan) using a lateral condensation method. The access cavity was sealed with Caviton®. The Pt did not undergo a radiograph at this appointment since she had to leave urgently.

Working length, apical size, and obturation technique

Canal	Working Length	Apical Size, Taper	Obturation Materials and Techniques
Single	19.0 mm	35, .04	Zinc oxide non-eugenol sealer, Lateral condensation

Post-Treatment Evaluation

Third visit (2-month follow-up): The Pt returned and reported that tooth #29 was free from symptoms. The numbness on the mental area had resolved and the tooth showed no tenderness to percussion, palpation, or biting, although the temporary restoration of the cervical area had been lost. PA radiography revealed that the root canal filling of tooth #29 was acceptable and the PARL of this tooth was reduced in size, although the cervical carious lesion had expanded (Figure 11.5). The tooth was scheduled for permanent restoration.

Fourth visit (15-month follow-up): At the postoperative (PO) evaluation, the Pt was asymptomatic and the tooth had been restored with a cast metal post and core, and a full metal crown. There was no tenderness to percussion, palpation, or biting. Radiographic examination revealed that tooth #29 showed a complete resolution of PARL (Figure 11.6A, B).

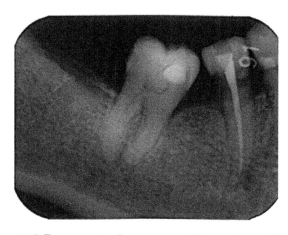

Figure 11.5 Two months after root canal filling of tooth #29.

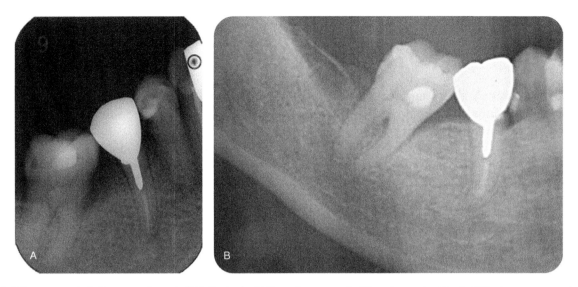

Figure 11.6 Fifteen-month follow-up of tooth #29. Periapical (A) and panoramic (B) radiographs. Tooth #29 shows a complete resolution of PARL.

Self-Study Questions

A. Describe the morphological characteristics and treatment considerations of the root canal system of mandibular premolars.

B. What are some advantages of the crown-down preparation technique?

C. Describe the anatomical relationship of the inferior alveolar nerve and mental foramen with mandibular premolars.

D. What are the causes of mental nerve paresthesia related to non-surgical endodontic treatment?

E. Explain clinical management of mental nerve paresthesia associated with endodontic infection and iatrogenic events related to endodontic treatment.

Answers to Self-Study Questions

A. Consistently high levels of success in endodontic treatment require an understanding of root canal anatomy and morphology. Mandibular premolars may present fairly simple root and root canal configuration, that is, single root/single canal without severe curvature. Nevertheless, mandibular premolars, particularly 1st premolars, may present with multiple roots and/or canals with considerable variations, making them challenging for endodontic treatment.

The frequency of single-canal mandibular premolars has been reported as 74–80.6% (1st premolars) and 88.4–97.5% (2nd premolars) (Zillich & Dowson 1973; Vertucci 1984; Calişkan *et al.* 1995). The pulp chamber of the single-canal mandibular premolar is usually oval and directed buccolingually. This shape may become round in the apical portion of the canal. However, it has been reported that the frequency of long-oval canals, where the long canal diameter is at least twice the short canal diameter, in single-canal mandibular premolars was 13% and 27% at 1–3 mm and 5 mm, respectively, from the apex (Wu *et al.* 2000). Instrumentation of the entire wall of long-oval canals can be difficult to achieve and a considerable portion of the canal wall can be uninstrumented (Versiani *et al.* 2013). Such recesses may harbor pulp remnants or bacterial biofilms, and thus may serve as potential sites of persistent intracanal infection. To disinfect the complexities associated with long-oval canals, meticulous irrigation using sonic/ultrasonic irrigation systems and apical negative pressure systems is recommended. One study has demonstrated that passive ultrasonic irrigation with sodium hypochlorite and a final rinse with chlorhexidine facilitates disinfection of *E. faecalis*-infected oval canals (Alves *et al.* 2011).

Mandibular premolars with multiple roots and root canals may present considerable morphological variations. In a study by Vertucci (1984), mandibular 1st premolars were classified as: one canal (70%); two canals joining at a common foramen (4%); two independent canals (1.5%); one canal bifurcating at the apex (24%); and two separate canals in two independent roots (0.5%). Mandibular 2nd premolars

are less variable; a single canal presents in 97.5%, and a canal that bifurcates at the apex in 2.5% (Vertucci 1984). Mandibular premolars with three canals (Figure 11.7A, B, C, D, E) or a C-shaped canal can also be found as rare variants.

Careful interpretation of preoperative radiographs is essential for providing insight into the number of existing root canals. In mandibular premolars with multiple roots and canals, the roots and canals may look unusual but the canals may not be evident in radiographs. Sudden narrowing or disappearance of the root canal space may indicate the presence of one or more extra canal(s). Radiographic appearance of the corresponding contralateral tooth may help in detecting additional canal(s), since bilateral teeth may present a similar morphology. Three-dimensional data obtained with cone beam-computed tomography (CBCT) is extremely useful in identifying the multiple-canal variants (Figure 11.7B).

The lingual canal of two-canal mandibular premolars may be difficult to locate, although direct access to the buccal canal may be readily possible. This is because the lingual canal often diverges from the buccal (main) canal at an acute angle. Thus, to facilitate the location of the lingual canal, the lingual wall of the access cavity should be extended lingually.

B. Crown-down preparation is classified as a coronal-to-apical preparation technique, where the preparation proceeds from coronal flaring to working length determination and apical preparation. This technique was originally advocated for handfile preparation as the "crown-down pressureless technique" (Morgan & Montgomery 1984) and has now been incorporated into various NiTi file systems.

With the crown-down technique, the coronal portion of the root canal system is first prepared mechanically using Gates–Glidden drills. The apical portion of the canal is then gradually approached sequentially with instruments of larger-to-smaller sizes until the apical constriction is reached. During this process, a fully cleaned and tapered canal space

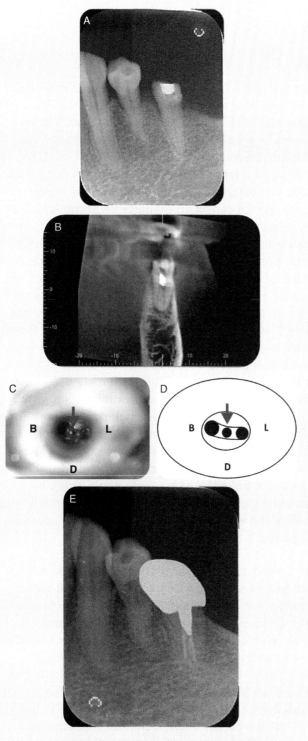

Figure 11.7 The case of tooth #20. (Not the case presented in this chapter; Courtesy Dr. Sonoko Noda, Tokyo Medical and Dental University) A: Preoperative periapical radiograph. B: Intraoperative CBCT (3DX, J. Morita, Kyoto, Japan). C: Microscopic view of canal orifices, showing the presence of three orifices. Arrow shows the orifice of the middle canal. D: Schematic drawing of C. E: Three months after root canal filling.

is left behind the preparation. The true working length is determined when the instrumentation reaches within 2–3 mm from the apical constriction (Morgan & Montgomery 1984).

The crown-down technique has several advantages over traditional apical-to-coronal preparation techniques such as standardized preparation and step-back technique. Early coronal flaring provides an "escape way" that reduces intracanal hydrostatic pressure generated in an apical direction. Early coronal flaring also facilitates penetration of irrigants into the root canal system and helps to create a fully cleaned coronal portion. For these reasons, the crown-down technique may provide less risk of apical extrusion of intracanal contents, i.e., bacteria, debris, dentin mud, and irrigant solution, which can cause postoperative flare-ups and delayed healing (Siqueira 2003). In the case presented, the primary reason for applying the crown-down preparation was to avoid postoperative flare-ups and the resulting exacerbation of paresthetic symptoms. Another advantage of the crown-down technique is that it provides less likelihood of working length shortening, which can occur during preparation of curved canals. This is because, in the crown-down technique, working length is determined after the achievement of straight-line access.

The crown-down technique is usually recommended in protocols for the use of NiTi rotary file systems in order to reduce the risk of intracanal instrument separation. Due to the presence of a space coronal to the site of preparation, the crown-down technique limits the binding of NiTi instruments to the root canal dentin, except in the apical flutes, and reduces torsional loads to the instruments during root canal preparation (Roland et al. 2002). In particular, this technique helps in reducing the risk of large torsional stress generation due to "taper lock," where a file is engaged into dentin over the length of its cutting blades and thus is at a great risk of fracture.

C. Knowledge of the spatial relationship between the inferior alveolar nerve and root apices is important in avoiding inadvertent nerve damage during endodontic procedures. This is because the inferior alveolar nerve is sensory, and thus its damage can cause disorders of sensory functions, such as numbness and neuropathic pain, which are uncommon, but serious, treatment complications.

After entering the mandibular canal through the mandibular foramen, the inferior alveolar nerve runs through the mandible body to the mental foramen, which is usually located in the premolar region. Within the mandible, the inferior alveolar nerve is located beneath the tooth roots and sometimes very close to the tooth apices. Although there are variations in the position of the nerve bundle in patients, mandibular 2nd premolars often show close proximity to the inferior alveolar nerve. In one study where human dried mandibles were used to measure the distance between the tooth apex and the mandibular canal, 2nd premolars and 2nd molars had the smallest distances, with a mean value of 4.7 mm and 3.7 mm, respectively (Denio, Torabinejad & Bakland 1992). Another study described how the inferior alveolar nerve rises to allow the mental branch to exit the mental foramen in the 2nd premolar area, which is associated with the proximity of the apex of this tooth type to the nerve (Knowles, Jergenson & Howard 2003). However, a recent study, where the distance was evaluated in CBCT images, described the apices of 2nd molars as being significantly closer to those of 2nd premolars and 1st molars (Kovisto, Ahmad & Bowles 2011).

The location of the mental foramen also needs to be considered when performing non-surgical as well as surgical endodontic therapy in mandibular premolars to avoid inadvertent neural damage. The mental foramen is an opening of the mandible and transmits the mental nerve, which is a branch of the posterior trunk of the inferior alveolar nerve and transmits the sensation from the buccal gingiva of the mandibular incisors, canine, and premolars, as well as the anterior aspects of the chin and lower lip. The foramen is usually located apical to the 2nd mandibular premolar or between the apices of the 1st and 2nd premolars, although it can be seen apical or mesial to the 1st premolar or distal to the 2nd premolar. A recent CBCT analysis showed that the root apex of the mandibular 2nd premolar (70%) was the closest to the mental foramen, followed by the 1st premolar (18%), and then the 1st molar (12%) (Chong et al. 2017). This study also described only

4% of root apices as being located within 3 mm from the mental foramen, with the position of the mental foramen being superior to the apices of the adjacent premolars in only 18% of cases (Chong et al. 2017). These findings may be associated with the fact that the incidence of paresthesia following endodontic treatment of mandibular premolars is low (0.96%) (Knowles et al. 2003). In addition, more than one mental foramen may be present; two mental foramina were noted in 1.8% (N = 110) of Asian skulls (Agthong, Huanmanop & Chentanez 2005). The additional foramina may be difficult to locate with panoramic and periapical films, but may be detected with CBCT scans.

Radiographic assessment of the mandibular canal and mental foramen is important for identification of the actual clinical location of the inferior alveolar nerve. However, radiographs must be interpreted cautiously, since these structures may not be clearly visible for several reasons, as will be discussed below. The mandibular canal is usually detected as a narrow radiolucent ribbon bordered by radio-opaque lines, although it may not always be a distinct bony-walled channel. In the anterior region, the canal wall is thinner, and thus less detectable on radiographs.

The advantages of panoramic radiography over periapical radiography in detecting the mandibular canal and mental foramen include the ability to view the entire body of the mandible. One study has shown that the detection rate of the mental foramen in panoramic radiographs was 94% (N = 545), although only 49% showed clear visibility (Jacobs et al. 2004). With respect to periapical radiographs, the detection rates of the mental foramen are smaller and have been reported to be 46.8% (N = 1000) in one study (Fishel et al. 1976), and 75% (N = 75) in another study (Phillips, Weller & Kulild 1990). In periapical films, the mental foramen sometimes mimics an inflammatory periapical lesion, particularly when the radiolucency is overlapping the apex of a premolar (Figure 11.8). In such a case, however, the mental foramen can be differentiated from pathologic conditions by its radiographic appearance, that is, better-maintained integrity of the lamina dura and periodontal ligament space. Exposures at different angulations are useful in the

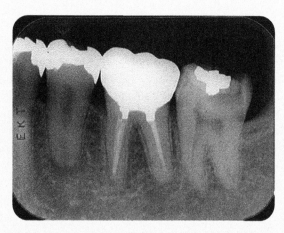

Figure 11.8 The case of tooth #20 (not the case presented in this chapter) showing a radiolucent area corresponding to the mental foramen around its apex.

differentiation, since the radiolucency representing the mental foramen moves from the apex by changing the angulation.

There are several reasons why the mandibular canal and the mental foramen are not always detectable in radiographs; these include difficulty in differentiating these structures from the trabecular pattern, and low radiographic contrast due to the thin mandibular bone or thick lingual cortical plate of the bone. In periapical films, these structures can be missed because of the narrower coverage, that is, when they are located out of the film edge.

The use of CBCT provides 3-D evaluation of the mandible, and its measurement accuracy is superior to panoramic and periapical radiographs. Thus, CBCT is currently the best available imaging technique to determine the accurate location of the mandibular canal and mental foramen (Aminoshariae, Su & Kulild 2014).

D. The overall incidence of mental nerve paresthesia is not clear, although one study reported that the incidence of paresthesia associated with non-surgical endodontic treatment of mandibular premolars was 0.96% (Knowles *et al.* 2003), indicating that such complication is fortunately uncommon.

Mental nerve paresthesia due to diseases of endodontic origin, that is, intracanal and periapical infection, is caused by several factors. One factor is mechanical pressure to the inferior alveolar nerve or mental nerve, which is associated with inflamma-

tory reaction; inflammatory edema formation and accumulation of purulent exudates may result in an increase in local pressure to a level sufficient to induce paresthesia. Nerve ischemia due to inflammation may also be a factor associated with paresthesia. A second factor is local production of bacterial metabolic products that are toxic to nerves.

Paresthesia is also a complication that is associated with endodontic treatment, and can be attributable to various causes (Ahonen & Tjäderhane 2011). Overinstrumentation and/or extrusion of endodontic materials into the vicinity of the inferior alveolar nerve or mental nerve are the major causes of mental nerve paresthesia. During chemomechanical root canal instrumentation, inadvertent extrusion of sodium hypochlorite can result in tissue necrosis due to the strong cytotoxicity and high tissue-dissolving activity of this solution, leading to pain, swelling, and possibly anesthesia of the mental nerve. Bacterial irritation can also occur during root canal instrumentation due to the extrusion of infected debris, which may also induce paresthesia by mechanisms similar to those induced by endodontic infection. Extruded calcium hydroxide intracanal medicament can also induce inferior alveolar nerve paresthesia (Ahlgren, Johannessen & Hellem 2003), possibly due to the causative potential of calcium hydroxide to induce inflammation and/or inhibition of nerve transmission by excessive calcium and hydroxide ions. Postoperative flare-ups following root canal instrumentation can be accompanied by mental nerve paresthesia, likely due to polietiological mechanisms, including bacterial, mechanical, and chemical irritation to the mental nerve (Morse 1997).

Overextruded root canal filling materials can induce paresthesis. Although gutta-percha is considered to be an inert root-filling material, overfilling of thermoplastic gutta-percha within the mandibular canal can generate paresthesia, likely due to thermal irritation and nerve compression. Another potential cause of paresthesia is root canal sealer, which can cause chemical irritation. In particular, zinc oxide and eugenol-based sealers show neurotoxic effects due to the action of eugenol, especially in the freshly mixed state. Paraformaldehyde-containing pastes are known to induce strong neurotoxic effects, and are not recommended for endodontic obturation.

E. The recovery potential of the nerve may be dependent on the extent of the damage and duration of the irritation, which show considerable variation among cases. Thus, paresthesia following transient nerve irritation, such as that induced by overinstrumentation, may resolve spontaneously within days or weeks. However, nerves suffering from prolonged damage due to chemical and mechanical irritation, such as that caused by gross overextension of neurotoxic materials, may not recover to the same degree (Ahonen & Tjäderhane 2011). In general, the first choice should be a more conservative treatment, including prescription of vitamin B12, which has the action of promoting peripheral nerve regeneration, and antibiotics to control infection. However, if surgical removal of foreign materials is deemed necessary, such as in the case of overextended neurotoxic material migrating along the mandibular nerve bundle, immediate surgical intervention, preferably within 48 hours, is recommended (Pogrel 2007).

Mental nerve paresthesia related to endodontic infection usually resolves after appropriate endodontic therapy in combination with drug therapy using antibiotics, corticosteroids, and/or vitamin B12 (Morse 1997). In the case presented, incision to establish drainage was effective for the resolution of symptoms related to acute inflammation, although great care should be taken not to damage the mental nerve during the incision. The decompression may have contributed, to a certain degree, to the recovery of sensation, whereas root canal therapy was necessary for the definitive resolution of the paresthetic symptoms. During the root canal therapy, great care should be taken to avoid iatrogenic events that could lead to the aggravation of paresthetic symptoms. In particular, postoperative acute exacerbation (flare-ups) following root canal instrumentation can be accompanied by mental nerve paresthesia (Morse 1997). Although acute exacerbation is caused by polietiological mechanisms, including bacterial, mechanical, and chemical irritation, and is often unpredictable, some procedures may have the potential to reduce the incidence of acute exacerbation. In this regard, instrumentation techniques with lesser amounts of apically extruded debris should be considered, such as the crown-down preparation technique, as discussed earlier. Copious and frequent irrigation is recommended since it can enhance the removal of canal contents such as infected dentin chips and microbial cells. Other possible measures include: completion of chemomechanical root canal preparation in one visit to remove maximum amount of irritants; correct measurement of the working length; and use of intracanal medicaments to facilitate microbial elimination (Siqueira 2003).

References

Agthong, S., Huanmanop, T. & Chentanez, V. (2005) Anatomical variations of the supraorbital, infraorbital, and mental foramina related to gender and side. *Journal of Oral and Maxillofacial Surgery* **63**, 800–804.

Ahlgren, F. K., Johannessen, A. C. & Hellem, S. (2003) Displaced calcium hydroxide paste causing inferior alveolar nerve paraesthesia: Report of a case. *Oral Surgery, Oral Medicine, Oral Pathology, Oral Radiology, and Endodontology* **96**, 734–737.

Ahonen, M. & Tjäderhane, L. (2011) Endodontic-related paresthesia: A case report and literature review. *Journal of Endodontics* **37**, 1460–1464.

Alves, F. R., Almeida, B. M., Neves, M. A. *et al.* (2011) Disinfecting oval-shaped root canals: Effectiveness of different supplementary approaches. *Journal of Endodontics* **37**, 496–501.

Aminoshariae, A., Su, A. & Kulild, J. C. (2014) Determination of the location of the mental foramen: A critical review. *Journal of Endodontics* **40**, 471–475.

Caliskan, M. K., Pehlivan, Y. Sepetçioğlu, F. *et al.* (1995) Root canal morphology of human permanent teeth in a Turkish population. *Journal of Endodontics* **21**, 200–204.

Chong, B. S., Gohil, K., Pawar, R. *et al.* (2017) Anatomical relationship between mental foramen, mandibular teeth and risk of nerve injury with endodontic treatment. *Clinical Oral Investigations* **21**, 381–387.

Denio, D., Torabinejad, M. & Bakland, L. (1992) Anatomical relationship of the mandibular canal to its surrounding structures in mature mandibles. *Journal of Endodontics* **18**, 161–165.

Fishel, D., Buchner, A., Hershkowith, A. *et al.* (1976) Roentgenologic study of the mental foramen. *Oral Surgery, Oral Medicine, Oral Pathology* **41**, 682–686.

Jacobs, R., Mraiwa, N., van Steenberghe, D. *et al.* (2004) Appearance of the mandibular incisive canal on panoramic radiographs. *Surgical and Radiologic Anatomy* **26**, 329–333.

Knowles, K. I., Jergenson, M. A. & Howard, J. H. (2003) Paresthesia associated with endodontic treatment of mandibular premolars. *Journal of Endodontics* **29**, 768–770.

Kovisto, T., Ahmad, M. & Bowles, W. R. (2011) Proximity of the mandibular canal to the tooth apex. *Journal of Endodontics* **37**, 311–315.

Morgan, L. F. & Montgomery, S. (1984) An evaluation of the crown-down pressureless technique. *Journal of Endodontics* **10**, 491–498.

Morse, D. R. (1997) Infection-related mental and inferior alveolar nerve paresthesia: Literature review and presentation of two cases. *Journal of Endodontics* **23**, 457–460.

Phillips, J. L., Weller, R. N. & Kulild, J. C. (1990) The mental foramen: 1. Size, orientation, and positional relationship to the mandibular second premolar. *Journal of Endodontics* **16**, 221–223.

Pogrel, M. A. (2007) Damage to the inferior alveolar nerve as the result of root canal therapy. *Journal of the American Dental Association* **138**, 65–69.

Roland, D. D., Andelin, W. E., Browning, D. F. *et al.* (2002) The effect of preflaring on the rates of separation for 0.04 taper nickel titanium rotary instruments. *Journal of Endodontics* **28**, 543–545.

Siqueira, J. F. Jr. (2003) Microbial causes of endodontic flare-ups. *International Endodontic Journal* **36**, 453–463.

Versiani, M. A., Leoni, G. B., Steier, L. *et al.* (2013) Micro-computed tomography study of oval-shaped canals prepared with the self-adjusting file, Reciproc, WaveOne, and ProTaper universal systems. *Journal of Endodontics* **39**, 1060–1066.

Vertucci, F. J. (1984) Root canal anatomy of the human permanent teeth. *Oral Surgery, Oral Medicine, Oral Pathology* **58**, 589–599.

Wu, M. K., R'oris, A., Barkis, D. et al. (2000) Prevalence and extent of long oval canals in the apical third. *Oral Surgery, Oral Medicine, Oral Pathology, Oral Radiology, and Endodontology* **89**, 739–743.

Zillich, R. & Dowson, J. (1973) Root canal morphology of mandibular first and second premolars. *Oral Surgery, Oral Medicine, Oral Pathology* **36**, 738–744.

12

Non-surgical Root Canal Treatment Case VI: Mandibular Premolar / Difficult Anatomy (three canals)

Savita Singh and Gayatri Vohra

LEARNING OBJECTIVES
- To demonstrate a thorough knowledge of the root and root canal morphology necessary to the success of non-surgical root canal therapy (NSRCT) for premolars.
- To understand how to prepare access to the mandibular premolar.
- To appreciate variations in root canal morphology in mandibular 1st and 2nd premolars and the different problems presented.
- To understand the importance of surrounding anatomical landmarks such as the mental foramen.

	Molars			Premolars		Canine	Incisors				Canine	Premolars		Molars		
							Maxillary arch									
Universal tooth designation system	1	2	3	4	5	6	7	8	9	10	11	12	13	14	15	16
International standards organization designation system	18	17	16	15	14	13	12	11	21	22	23	24	25	26	27	28
Palmer method	8	7	6	5	4	3	2	1	1	2	3	4	5	6	7	8
Palmer method	8	7	6	5	4	3	2	1	1	2	3	4	5	6	7	8
International standards organization designation system	48	47	46	45	44	43	42	41	31	32	33	34	35	36	37	38
Universal tooth designation system	32	31	30	29	28	27	26	25	24	23	22	21	20	19	18	17
							Mandibular arch									
	Right									**Left**						

Clinical Cases in Endodontics, First Edition. Edited by Takashi Komabayashi.
© 2018 John Wiley & Sons, Inc. Published 2018 by John Wiley & Sons, Inc.

Chief Complaint

"I have been having discomfort on and off for past few days. Especially, cold has been bothering."

Medical History

The patient (Pt) was a 64-year-old male. He had high blood pressure (BP), which was under control, and took Arenol, 50 mg daily for this condition. Pt had allergy to penicillin. No significant findings were noted as a result of complete review of systems. No contraindications to dental treatment were identified.

The Pt was classified as American Society of Anesthesiologists Physical Scale Status (ASA) Class II.

Dental History

Tooth #21 had a cervical composite restoration. The Pt had been having discomfort for the previous month, mild to begin with but later when he drank cold water or went for a walk, he could feel cold sensitivity on the tooth. It bothered him and was painful. There was no discomfort with hot beverage. Tooth #20 also had a cervical composite restoration.

Clinical Examination (Diagnostic Procedures)
Examinations
Extra-Oral Examination (EOE)

There was no swelling present and no tenderness on palpation, especially in the area around tooth #21.

Intra-Oral Examination (IOE)

Examination showed that probing depth of tooth #21 was within normal limits such as MB 3 mm, B 2 mm, DB 3 mm, ML 3 mm, L 2 mm, DL 3 mm.

Diagnostic Tests

Tooth	#22	#21	#20
Percussion	–	+	–
Palpation	-	-	-
Cold	+	++	+
Tooth Slooth	–	–	–

++: Exaggerated response to cold; +: Response to percussion and normal response to cold; -: No response to percussion, palpation, and tooth slooth

Radiographic Findings

Two radiographs were taken, straight (Figure 12.1A) and mesial-angled (Figure 12.1B). They showed tooth #21 and tooth #20 had cervical composite restoration; the periapical areas seemed to be normal. The root had unusual anatomy; it was very wide and showed trifurcation of the canal system.

Pretreatment Diagnosis
Pulpal

Symptomatic Irreversible Pulpitis, tooth #21

Apical

Symptomatic Apical Periodontitis, tooth #21

Treatment Plan
Recommended

Emergency: None
Definitive: Non-surgical root canal treatment (NSRCT)

Alternative

Extraction or no treatment

Restorative

Crown

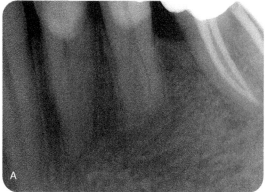
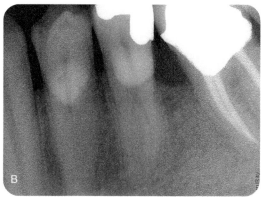

Figure 12.1 Preoperative radiographs of tooth #21, showing Class 5 restoration and wide root tri-furcating at coronal-middle third of root. A: Straight view; B: Mesial angled view.

Prognosis

Favorable	Questionable	Unfavorable
X		

But will depend upon successfully finding and obturating all the canals

Clinical Procedures: Treatment Record

First Visit (Day 1): Pt's BP was 130/76 mmHg. Anesthesia was achieved with 2% lidocaine (lido) with 1:100,000 epinephrine (epi) (1 carpule), left Inferior alveolar nerve block (IANB), 1 carpule of 2% lido with 1:100,000 epi infiltration around the tooth. The treatment was performed using a Zeiss microscope (OPMI-Pico, Carl Zeiss-USA, Dublin, CA, USA). Tooth #21 was clamped and a rubber dam (RD) placed. Access was made using No. #4 round carbide bur. The tooth was dis-occluded and the access was widened with a long-fissure bur. The shape of the access was oval but made little wider mesial–distally (MD) due to an unusual trifurcated anatomy of the root. On entry into the pulp chamber, one main canal orifice was found which split into three different canal orifices at the coronal–mid-root level. Mesio-buccal (MB), Disto-buccal (DB) and Lingual (L) canals were identified with magnification and illumination. Gates Glidden drills #3, #2, and, #1 with a brushing motion were used in a crown-down fashion to enlarge the main orifice to the level of the trifurcation to obtain straight line access to all the three canals. MB, DB and L canals were located, and their orifices were widened using S1 and S2 ProTaper® Universal files (Dentsply Sirona, Ballaigues, Switzerland). Full-strength sodium hypochlorite (6 % NaOCl) was used for canal irrigation. Canals were dried with paper points (PPs). A size #10 K-file (ReadySteel® K-File, Dentsply Sirona, Ballaigues, Switzerland) was pre-curved and used to determine the working length of the canals, together with an electric apex locator (Root ZX®II, J. Morita, Kyoto, Japan). All canals measured 21 mm in length. Biomechanical preparation was started. Canals were hand-instrumented to working length with size #15 K-file (ReadySteel® K-File, Dentsply Sirona, Ballaigues, Switzerland). Canals were irrigated with 6 % NaOCl and then dried with PPs. After drying the canals, Calcium hydroxide (Ca(OH)$_2$ MultiCal™, Watertown, MA, USA) was placed inside the canal, cotton pellet (CP) and Cavit™ (3M, Two Harbors, MN, USA) and Fuji IX GP® (GC America Inc., Alsip, IL, USA) was

placed for temporalization. Pt was advised to take 200 mg to 400 mg of Ibuprofen every 4–6 hours as needed for any post-operative (PO) discomfort and inflammation.

Second Visit (3 week): Pt was doing well, with no discomfort or changes in medical history. BP was recorded at 128/72 mmHg. 2% lido with 1:100,000 epi (1 carpule) as left IANB and 1 carpule of 2% lido with 1: 100,000 epi infiltration around the tooth were administered. A RD was placed and temporary cement was removed using a round bur. Irrigation was done using 6% NaOCl, and biomechanical instrumentation was completed in all three canals. All the canals were enlarged to size #25/ .04 taper of ProFile® (Dentsply Sirona, Ballaigues, Switzerland), the canals were dried using PPs, and a periapical (PA) radiograph was taken with gutta-percha (GP) in DB and L canal. First, the DB and L canals were obturated and then the third canal was obturated (Figure 12.2). System-B™ (Kerr, Orange, CA, USA) and Obtura™ system (Spartan Obtura, Algonquin, IL, USA) was used for obturation by continuous-wave technique. The GP in each canal was seared 4–5 mm from the apex and then backfilled with Obtura™ system. After obturating the DB and L canal, a GP cone was placed in MB canal and a PA radiograph was taken (Figure 12.3). The MB canal was then obturated (Figure 12.4). Size #25/ .04 taper Lexicon® GP point (Dentsply Sirona, Johnson City, TN, USA) and Pulp Canal Sealer™ EWT (Kerr Endodontic) were used. CP, Cavit™, and Fuji IX GP® was placed. Post-obturation radiographs were taken (Figure 12.5A, B). Post-operative instructions (POI) were given. The Pt was instructed to take over-the-counter ibuprofen 200 mg to 400 mg every 4–6 hours as needed for post-operative discomfort. The Pt was advised to get a crown.

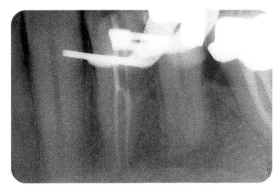

Figure 12.2 Down-packed and backfilled DB and L canals and checking the MB canal.

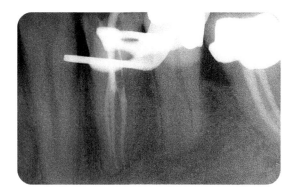

Figure 12.3 Checking the MB canal.

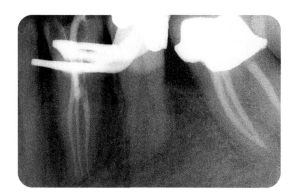

Figure 12.4 The MB canal obturated.

Working length, apical size, and obturation technique

Canal	Working Length	Apical Size, Taper	Obturation Materials and Techniques
MB	21.0 mm	25, .04	Pulp Canal Sealer™ EWT, Continuous wave
L	21.0 mm	25, .04	Pulp Canal Sealer™ EWT, Continuous wave
DB	21.0 mm	25, .04	Pulp Canal Sealer™ EWT, Continuous wave

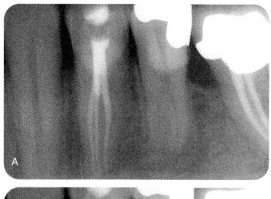

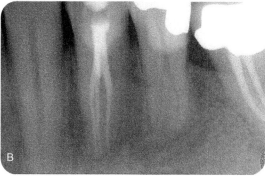

Figure 12.5 A: Postobturation radiograph showing three canals with three different exit portals; B: Postobturation radiograph showing three exit portals.

If cone beam-computed tomography (CBCT) had been available, it would have been beneficial to give a three-dimensional view of the tooth.

Post-Treatment Evaluation

There were no post-treatment evaluations as Pt moved out of the country.

Self-Study Questions

A. What are the probabilities of bifurcation of mandibular 1st premolars?

B. What are the anatomical and morphological factors to consider before non-surgical treatment of mandibular premolars?

C. Why is proper imaging important before treating mandibular premolars?

D. What are the essential steps to be taken to successfully treat mandibular premolars?

E. What are the potential consequences of over instrumentation and/or apical sealer extrusion on a mandibular premolar?

Answers to Self-Study Questions

A. Root canal morphology is unique to each individual tooth. It has been shown to be variable to different genders as well as races (Caliskan *et al.* 1995).

The clinician must be familiar with various pathways root canals take to the apex. The pulp canal system is complex, and canals may branch, divide, and rejoin. Weine (1996) has categorized the root canal systems in any root in four basic types and Vertucci (1984) identified eight pulp space configurations.

Mandibular 1st premolars in particular are known to have complex root canal anatomy, which can make diagnosing and treating the pulp canal space challenging. A good clinician must know the probabilities of additional pulp canal spaces in any given tooth before proceeding with the treatment. According to a study on root canal configuration of the mandibular 1st premolar (Baisden, Kulild & Weller 1992), the incidence of one root canal system varied from 69.3 to 86%; two canals, 14 to 25.5%; and three canals, 0.4 to 0.9%.

B. There are several factors that should be considered, such as gender, race, and position of the tooth in relation to other teeth (Caliskan *et al.* 1995). In addition, there are certain anatomical factors that are of unique importance to the premolars: (1) position of the inferior alveolar nerve (IAN) in relation to the apex of the tooth; (2) presence or absence of a cortical tunnel around the IAN; and (3) buccolingual and mesiodistal dimension of the root canal system.

- *Position of the IAN*: Before undertaking procedures on mandibular premolars, it is critical to know the location of the IAN with respect to the surrounding structures to avoid injury. According to Denio, Torabinejad & Bakland (1992), the IAN canal is located buccal to the 2nd molar, lingual to the 1st molar and directly inferior to the 2nd premolar.

- *Presence or absence of a cortical tunnel around the IAN*: The mandibular canals appear in some cases as distinct bony-walled channels within porous lined trabecular bone. However, in many cases the canals have no definite borders apical to the 1st molars and 2nd premolars (Denio *et al.*1992). Olivier (1927) as well as Carter and

Keen (1971), found that 60% of mandible specimens contained canals while 40% of the dissections had no distinct canals. These findings suggest that the clinician should identify the canal position and proceed with caution while treating the mandibular premolar.

- *Buccolingual and mesiodistal dimension of the root canal system*: Non-surgical treatment of mandibular premolar tooth may pose a challenge to the most skilled clinician. These groups of teeth tend to have a high flare-up and failure rate. The root canal system of mandibular 1st premolars tends to be wider buccolingually than mesiodistally. If two canals are present, direct access to the buccal canal is usually possible; however, extension of lingual access may be necessary to gain access to the lingual canal (Walton & Torabinejad 1996).

C. A proper imaging report, and a proper understanding of the image report, are of paramount importance for a good clinical outcome. Images that can be helpful for treatment of a mandibular premolar include intra-operative periapical radiograph with mesial and distal angles, and CBCT. One good hint of the probability of more than one canal or an accessory canal would be the disappearance of a pulp canal midway of the root or at a certain level apically. The prudent decision to follow upon seeing this would be to take multiple-angled intra-oral periapical radiographs or a CBCT. The imaging would help the clinician to decide at what distance he/she should look for the additional canal, as well as allow him/her to stay away from danger zones such as the furcation areas, and to detect the presence and severity of concavity of distal surface. Evaluation of CBCT images results in identification of a greater number of root canal systems (Matherne *et al.* 2008).

D. Cleaning and shaping of the root canal system is a precursor to a well-obturated and sealed canal, which would be a stepping stone to the longevity and long-term health of the tooth. Cleaning of the root canal system would include identifying all the canals within the root canal system, and accurately measuring and shaping with a reliable rotary system. Taking these steps will provide the clinician with an area that can be well obturated and sealed three-dimensionally. Knowledge of both basic root and root canal morphology as well as possible variation in the anatomy of the root canal system is important to achieve success in non-surgical root canal treatment (Cleghorn, Christie & Dong 2007). Ingle (1961) reported that the most significant cause of endodontic failures was incomplete canal instrumentation, followed by incorrect canal obturation. Slowey (1979) has indicated that, probably because of the variations in canal anatomy, the mandibular premolars are the most difficult teeth to treat endodontically. Another step that would aid the clinician in treatment would be the addition of a microscope in the armamentarium for better visualization. Tactile sense with a fine, curved stainless steel file is also often the best guide to the detection of the accessory canal systems (England, Hartwell & Lance 1991).

E. Root canal treatment of the mandibular premolar presents unique challenges due to its proximity to the IAN canal. Three-dimensional obturation of the root canal system constitutes one of the goals of endodontic treatment. Ideally, the filling material should be confined to the root canal space without extending to periapical tissues or other neighboring structures (Himel & DiFiore 2009; Gonzalez-Martin et al. 2010). However, if filling materials are accidentally extruded to neighboring neurovascular structures, nerve injury, with an ensuing altered sensation, may occur (Rosen et al. 2016). Endodontic therapy might also damage the IAN. Several mechanisms have been proposed to explain this damage, including neurotoxic effect from root canal filling material penetrating the IAN (Escoda-Francoli et al. 2007; Pogrel 2007); mechanical pressure on the nerve caused by over-extension of filling material or over-instrumentation with hand or rotary files; or an increase in temperature proximal to the IAN greater than 10° C (Escoda-Francoli et al. 2007). IAN damage has been suggested to occur in 1% of mandibular premolars that receive root canal treatment (Escoda-Francoli et al. 2007).

References

Baisden, M.K., Kulild, J.C. & Weller, R.N. (1992) Root canal configuration of the mandibular first premolar. *Journal of Endodontics* **18**, 505–508.

Caliskan M.K., Pehlivan. Y. Sepetcioqlu F. *et al.* (1995) Root canal morphology of human permanent teeth in a Turkish population. *Journal of Endodontics* **21**, 200–204.

Carter, R.B. & Keen, E.N. (1971) The intramandibular course of the inferior alveolar nerve. *Journal of Anatomy* **106**, 433–440.

Cleghorn, B.M., Christie, W.H. & Dong, C.C. (2007) The root and root canal morphology of the human mandibular first premolar: a literature review. *Journal of Endodontics* **33**, 509–516.

Denio, D., Torabinejad, M. & Bakland, L. K. (1992) Anatomical relationship of the mandibular canal to its surrounding structures in mature mandibles. *Journal of Endodontics* **18**, 161–165.

England, M. C., Hartwell, G. R. & Lance, J. R. (1991) Detection and treatment of multiple canals in mandibular premolars. *Journal of Endodontics* **17**, 174–178.

Escoda-Francoli, J., Canalda-Sahli C., Soler, A. *et al.* (2007) Inferior alveolar nerve damage because of overextended endodontic material: a problem of sealer cement biocompatibility? *Journal of Endodontics* **33**, 1484–1489.

Gonzalez-Martin, M., Torres-Lagares, D., Gutierrez-Perez, J. L. et al. (2010) Inferior alveolar nerve paresthesia after overfilling of endodontic sealer into the mandibular canal. *Journal of Endodontics* **36**, 1419–1421.

Himel, V. T. & DiFiore, P. M. (2009) Obturation of root canal systems. *Endodontics: Colleagues for Excellence Newsletter.* Chicago: American Association of Endodontists.

Ingle, J. I. (1961) A standardized endodontic technique utilizing newly designed instruments and filling materials. *Oral Surgery, Oral Medicine, Oral Pathology* **14**, 83–91.

Matherne, R. P., Angelopolous, C., Kulild, J. C. et al. (2008) Use of cone-beam computed tomography to identify root canal systems in vitro. *Journal of Endodontics* **34**, 87–89.

Olivier, E. (1927) The inferior dental canal and its nerve in the adult. *British Dental Journal* **49**, 356–358.

Pogrel, M. A. (2007) Damage to the inferior alveolar nerve as the result of root canal therapy. *Journal of the American Dental Association* **138**, 65–69.

Rosen, E., Goldberger, T., Taschieri, D. *et al.* (2016) The prognosis of altered sensation after extrusion of root canal filling materials: a systematic review of the literature. *Journal of Endodontics* **42**, 873–879.

Slowey, R. R. (1979) Root canal anatomy. Road map to successful endodontics. *Dental Clinics of North America* **23**, 555–573.

Vertucci, F. J. (1984) Root canal anatomy of the human permanent teeth. *Oral Surgery, Oral Medicine, Oral Pathology* **58**, 589–599.

Walton, R. & Torabinejad, M. (1996) *Principles and practice of endodontics.* 2nd edn. Philadelphia: WB Saunders.

Weine, F. S. (1996) *Endodontic Therapy*, 5th edn, p. 243. St. Louis, MO: Mosby-Yearbook.

13

Non-surgical Root Canal Treatment Case VII: Maxillary Molar/Four Canals (MB1, MB2, DB, P)

Khaled Seifelnasr

LEARNING OBJECTIVES

■ To identify normal anatomy for the maxillary 1st and 2nd molars.

■ To identify and understand the prevalence of the second mesiobuccal canal in maxillary molars.

■ To understand the location of second mesiobuccal canals in maxillary molars.

	Molars			Premolars		Canine	Incisors				Canine	Premolars		Molars		
							Maxillary arch									
Universal tooth designation system	1	2	3	4	5	6	7	8	9	10	11	12	13	14	15	16
International standards organization designation system	18	17	16	15	14	13	12	11	21	22	23	24	25	26	27	28
Palmer method	8⌋	7⌋	6⌋	5⌋	4⌋	3⌋	2⌋	1⌋	⌊1	⌊2	⌊3	⌊4	⌊5	⌊6	⌊7	⌊8
Palmer method	8⌉	7⌉	6⌉	5⌉	4⌉	3⌉	2⌉	1⌉	⌈1	⌈2	⌈3	⌈4	⌈5	⌈6	⌈7	⌈8
International standards organization designation system	48	47	46	45	44	43	42	41	31	32	33	34	35	36	37	38
Universal tooth designation system	32	31	30	29	28	27	26	25	24	23	22	21	20	19	18	17
							Mandibular arch									
			Right									**Left**				

Clinical Cases in Endodontics, First Edition. Edited by Takashi Komabayashi.
© 2018 John Wiley & Sons, Inc. Published 2018 by John Wiley & Sons, Inc.

Chief Complaint

"I have severe pain in the left side of my face, I feel it throbbing sometimes. I'm not sure where the pain is coming from."

Medical History

The patient (Pt) was a 37-year-old white female. Her vital signs were as follows: blood pressure (BP) 118/72 mmHg; pulse, 74 beats per minute and regular; respiratory rate, 18 breaths per minute. A complete review of systems was conducted. No significant findings were noted. There were no contraindications to dental treatment (Tx).

The Pt was American Society of Anesthesiologists Physical Status Scale (ASA) Class I.

Dental History

The Pt had extensive restorative Tx. Teeth #12, #14, and #15 were observed to have large restorations. She was referred by her general dentist for evaluation of symptoms and Tx.

Clinical Evaluation (Diagnostic Procedures)
Examinations
Extra-oral Examination (EOE)

EOE revealed no significant findings, and no lymphaneopathy or extra-oral swellings were noted. The temporomandibular joint (TMJ) demonstrated no discomfort to opening or closing, no popping, clicking, or deviation to either side upon opening.

Intra-oral Examination (IOE)

IOE revealed multiple extensive restorations.

Diagnostic Tests

Tooth	#13	#14	#15
Percussion	–	+	–
Palpation	–	–	–
Thermal	Normal vital	Non–vital	Normal vital

+: Pain/response; –: No pain/no response

Radiographic Findings

Periapical (PA) radiographic findings revealed large restorations invloving multiple surfaces of teeth #12, #14, and #15 (Figure 13.1). Tooth #14 showed a large composite restoration in close proximity to the pulp. The palatal root of tooth #14 showed apical resorption with a well defined radiolucent lesion involving the apex of that root.

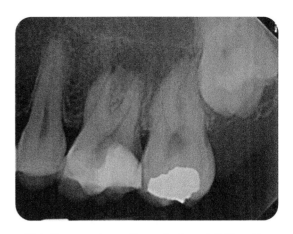

Figure 13.1 Preoperative radiograph, first visit (Day 1).

Pretreatment Diagnosis
Pulpal

Necrotic Pulp, tooth #14

Apical

Symptomatic Apical Periodontitis, tooth #14

Treatment Plan

Emergency: None

Definitive: Non-surgical Root Canal Treatment (NSRCT) of tooth #14

Alternative

Extraction or no treatment

Restorative

Core build-up and full coverage restoration

Prognosis

Favorable	Questionable	Unfavorable
X		

Clinical Procedures: Treatment Record

First visit (Day 1): A review of medical history (RMHX) of Pt was conducted. Informed consent, written and verbal, was obtained. A local infiltration was performed with 72 mg of 2% Xylocaine® with 1:100,000 epinephrine (epi). A rubber dam (RD) was placed and an access was made through the occlusal surface of the tooth. The pulp chamber was irrigated with 2.5% sodium hypochlorite (NaOCl); four canal orifices were located. A necrotic pulp was noted upon access. Working-length measurements were taken radiographically and verified via an electronic apex

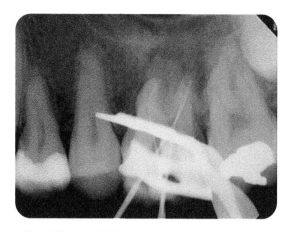

Figure 13.2 MB1 and DB length-estimation radiograph (Day 1).

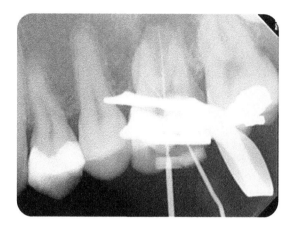

Figure 13.3 MB2 and P length-estimation radiograph (Day 1).

locator (Root ZX® II, J. Morita, Kyoto, Japan) (Figures 13.2 and 13.3). All canals were instrumented using .04 taper Vortex® Nickel Titanium (NiTi) rotary files (Dentsply Sirona, Johnson City, TN, USA). 2.5% NaOCl, 17% ethylenediaminetetraacetic acid (EDTA), and RC-Prep® were utilized throughout the procedure. Mesio-Buccal (MB) 1 and MB 2 canals were enlarged to a size #30, .04 taper, the Disto-Buccal (DB) canal was enlarged to a size #35, 0.04 taper, and the Palatal canal was enlarged to a size #60, .04 taper. The irrigants were then introduced to the canals after cleaning and shaping, followed by activation via ultrasonic activation files. All canals were dried with sterile paper points and medicated with calcium hydroxide ($Ca(OH)_2$) powder freshly mixed with sterile saline. The $Ca(OH)_2$ paste was packed and distributed throughout the canals. The access was closed with a sterile dry cotton pellet and Cavit™ (3M, Two Harbors, MN, USA). Occlusion was

verified. Oral and written postoperative instructions were given.

Second visit (Day 2): Pt was contacted for postoperative follow-up; the Pt reported that the dull pain had subsided and that she was feeling well.

Third visit (Day 14): RMHX; no changes were noted. Local infiltration with 72 mg of 2% Xylocaine with 1:100,000 epi was administered. A RD was placed and access was made through the Cavit™. The pulp chamber was irrigated with 2.5% NaOCl and 17% EDTA. Ultrasonic files were utilized to remove the $Ca(OH)_2$ and the final rotary instruments were reintroduced in the canals to the previous diameters and working distances. All canals were dried with sterile paper points and obturated with gutta-percha (GP) and AH Plus® Root Canal Sealer (Dentsply Sirona, Konstanz, Germany) utilizing the warm vertical condensation technique. A radiograph was taken (Figure 13.4).

Working length, apical size, and obturation technique

Canal	Working Length	Apical Size, Taper	Obturation Material and Techniques
MB1	19.5 mm	30, .04	GP, AH Plus® sealer Warm vertical condensation
MB2	19.0 mm	30, .04	GP, AH Plus® sealer Warm vertical condensation
DB	19.5 mm	35, .04	GP, AH Plus® sealer Warm vertical condensation
P	20.0 mm	60, .04	GP, AH Plus® sealer Warm vertical condensation

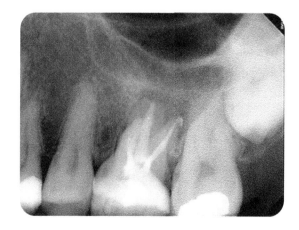

Figure 13.4 Postoperative radiograph, second visit (Day 14).

Postoperative Evaluation

Fourth visit (15-month follow-up): Pt reported she had been asymptomatic. Soft tissues appeared to be normal and tooth had no apical tenderness or

percussion sensitivity. PA radiograph demonstrated a healed tooth #14 with intact lamina dura (Figure 13.5).

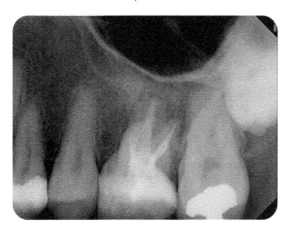

Figure 13.5 One-year follow-up radiograph showing healed lesion.

Figure 13.6 illustrates the location of MB2 intra-orally for the case.

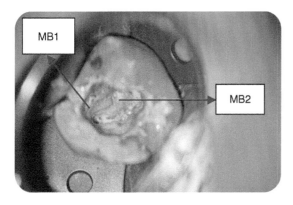

Figure 13.6 Intra-oral picture showing location of MB2 (Day 14).

Figures 13.7 to 13.11 illustrate the prevalence of MB2 in maxillary molars.

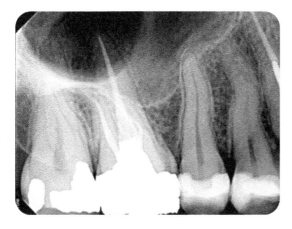

Figure 13.7 Maxillary 1st molar tooth #3 showing presence of MB2.

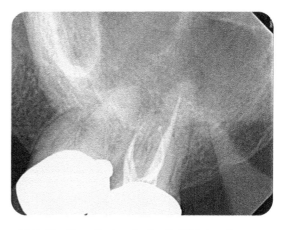

Figure 13.8 Maxillary 2nd molar tooth #15 showing presence of MB2.

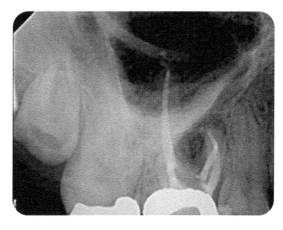

Figure 13.9 Maxillary 1st molar tooth #3 showing presence of MB2.

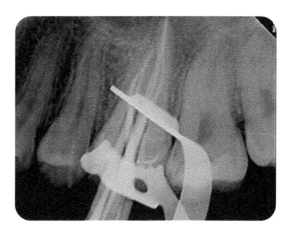

Figure 13.10 Maxillary 1st molar tooth #14 showing presence of MB2.

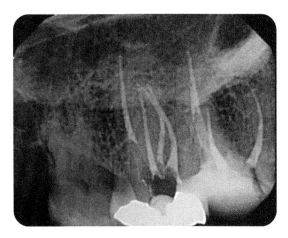

Figure 13.11 Maxillary 2nd molar tooth #2 showing presence of MB2.

Figures 13.12 and 13.13 illustrate the unusual anatomy of maxillary molars.

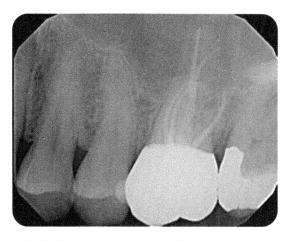

Figure 13.13 Maxillary molar tooth #14 with the second palatal canal and MB2.

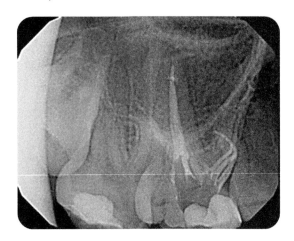

Figure 13.12 Unusual Maxillary 1st molar, tooth #3, showing presence of MB1, MB2 and MB3.

Self-Study Questions

A. According to most root anatomy studies, how many roots do the maxillary 1st and 2nd molars have?

B. What is the most common cause for non-surgical root canal treatment failure of maxillary molars?

C. What is the average prevalence of a second mesiobuccal canal in maxillary 1st molars?

D. What is the average prevalence of a second mesiobuccal canal in maxillary 2nd molars?

E. What tools can a clinician utilize to locate the second mesiobuccal canal in maxillary molars?

Answers to Self-Study Questions

A. The maxillary 1st and 2nd molars most commonly have three roots, a mesiobuccal root, a distobuccal root, and a palatal root. The internal anatomy of those roots is highly variable, especially in the mesiobuccal root. The mesiobuccal root of maxillary molars tends to have two canals, with maxillary 1st molars tending to have a higher prevalence of two canals in the mesiobuccal root than maxillary 2nd molars (Cleghorn, Christie & Dong 2006).

B. The most common cause for non-surgical root canal failure is failure to locate and treat the second mesiobuccal canal in maxillary 1st and 2nd molars. Studies have shown that failure to locate and properly treat second mesiobuccal canals in maxillary molars will affect the long term prognosis and success of these teeth, and will eventually lead to endodontic failure (Wolcott *et al.* 2005); therefore, it is crucial for the clinician to be knowledgeable and thorough when treating maxillary molars.

C and **D.** There have been multiple studies that have examined and evaluated the presence of a second mesiobuccal canal in maxillary molars. According to an *in vitro* study, a second mesiobuccal canal was found in up to 95.2% of both 1st and second maxillary molars (Kulild & Peters 1990). Other studies evaluated clinical existence of a second mesiobuccal canal in 1st maxillary molars and found it to be present in 71.2% of the time (Fogel, Peikoff & Christie 1994). Another interesting study, which was conducted over a period of 8 years, found that initially the clinician located a second mesiobuccal canal in 73.2% for 1st molars and 50.7% for 2nd molars. However, when the clinician gained more experience and utilized a dental operating microscope, the mesiobuccal canal was found in 93% and 60.4% for 1st and 2nd molars, respectively (Stropko 1999). A more advanced study reviewed 34 studies and weighted the average of a total of 8,399 1st molars, concluding that a second mesiobuccal canal was present in 56.8%. The study further found that the distal root and the palatal root had one canal in 98.3% and 99% respectively (Cleghorn *et al.* 2006).

E. A wise and properly trained clinician would realize that the prevalence of a second mesiobuccal canal is high and should utilize dental technological advancements such as the dental operating microscope, piezo ultrasonics, and specialty burs to aid in finding these canals.

References

Cleghorn, B. M., Christie, W. H. & Dong, C. C. (2006) Root and root canal morphology of the human permanent maxillary first molar: A literature review. *Journal of Endodontics* **32**, 813–821.

Fogel, H. M., Peikoff, M. D. & Christie, W. H. (1994) Canal configuration in the mesiobuccal root of the maxillary first molar: A clinical study. *Journal of Endodontics* **20**, 135–137.

Kulild, J. C. & Peters, D. D. (1990) Incidence and configuration of canal systems in the mesiobuccal root of maxillary first and second molars. *Journal of Endodontics* **16**, 311–317.

Stropko, J. J. (1999) Canal morphology of maxillary molars: Clinical observations of canal configurations. *Journal of Endodontics* **25**, 446–450.

Wolcott, J., Ishley, D., Kennedy, W. *et al.* (2005) A 5 yr clinical investigation of second mesiobuccal canals in endodontically treated and retreated maxillary molars. *Journal of Endodontics* **31**, 262–264.

14

Non-surgical Root Canal Treatment Case VIII: Mandibular Molar

Ahmed O Jamleh and Nada Ibrahim

LEARNING OBJECTIVES
- To understand the correct questions for obtaining an adequate history of presenting symptoms.
- To be able to form a diagnosis of pulpal and periapical conditions based on complete data from history, examination, and tests.
- To be able to manage pulpal and periapical diseases conservatively by nonsurgical root canal treatment.

- To recognize that effective root canal debridement is necessary to attain complete resolution of a draining sinus.
- To describe the clinical and radiographic criteria used to determine success of nonsurgical root canal treatment.

	Molars			Premolars		Canine	Incisors				Canine	Premolars		Molars		
							Maxillary arch									
Universal tooth designation system	1	2	3	4	5	6	7	8	9	10	11	12	13	14	15	16
International standards organization designation system	18	17	16	15	14	13	12	11	21	22	23	24	25	26	27	28
Palmer method	8	7	6	5	4	3	2	1	1	2	3	4	5	6	7	8
Palmer method	8	7	6	5	4	3	2	1	1	2	3	4	5	6	7	8
International standards organization designation system	48	47	46	45	44	43	42	41	31	32	33	34	35	36	37	38
Universal tooth designation system	32	31	30	29	28	27	26	25	24	23	22	21	20	19	18	17
							Mandibular arch									
	Right										**Left**					

Chief Complaint

"I have a pimple on the left side of my face that oozes intermittently."

Medical History

The patient (Pt) was a 9-year-old male. He had normal mental and physical development, and normal vital signs at presentation (height 146 cm; weight 55 kg; vital signs were as follows: blood pressure (BP) 117/53 mmHg, right arm seated; pulse 94 beats per minute (BPM) and regular; respiratory rate (RR) 18 breaths per minute; temperature 36.6°C). His past medical history was unremarkable with no known drug allergies (NKDA). He used no medications apart from an antibiotic, recently prescribed by his dermatologist, to treat a draining sinus on his face, which apparently failed to respond.

The Pt was considered American Society of Anesthesiologists Physical Status Scale (ASA) Class I.

Dental History

A few months ago, the Pt was referred to a primary care dental clinic and had tooth #19 accessed with partial root canal instrumentation and non-setting calcium hydroxide paste (Ca(OH)$_2$; UltraCal® XS; Ultradent, South Jordan, UT, USA) placement. The dentist referred him to the endodontic clinic for further management.

Clinical Evaluation (Diagnostic Procedures)
Examinations
Extra-oral Examination (EOE)

EOE showed a 1 cm erythematous nodule at the skin overlying the left mandibular body (Figure 14.1A). The nodule had a crusted surface and was tender to touch. There was no fever, facial swelling, or cervical lymphadenopathy.

Intra-oral Examination (IOE)

IOE revealed poor oral hygiene and chronically inflamed gingivae. Tooth #19 was temporarily restored with resin modified glass ionomer dental filling (RMGI) (Photac™ Fil, 3M ESPE, Neuss, Germany; Figure 14.1B), exhibited no mobility or periodontal pocketing, and had fairly intact margins. The tooth was non-responsive to cold test or electric pulp stimulation test, but was not tender to percussion and palpation.

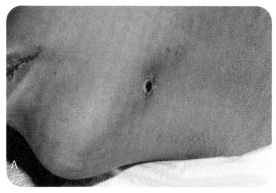
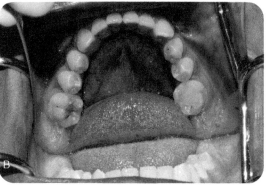

Figure 14.1 Preoperative images showing a 1 cm erythematous and crusted-surface nodule (A) and the offending tooth with no intraoral swelling (B).

Diagnostic Tests

Tooth	#18	#19	#20	#30 (Contralateral)
Percussion	–	–	–	–
Palpation	–	–	–	–
Cold	+	–	+	+
Mobility	WNL	WNL	WNL	WNL
EPT	+	–	+	+

EPT: Electric pulp test; WNL: Within normal limits; +: Responsive; –: Not responsive

Radiographic Findings

A periapical (PA) radiograph showed a radiolucency involving the mesial (M) root apex and extending to the furcation area. The lamina dura surrounding the M root was lost with no evidence of external or internal root resorption (Figure 14.2).

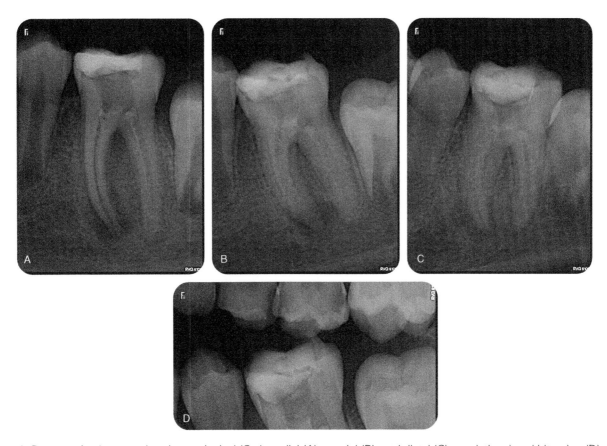

Figure 14.2 Preoperative images showing periapical (Orthoradial (A), mesial (B), and distal (C) angulations) and bitewing (D) radiographs.

Pretreatment Diagnosis
Pulpal
Previously initiated therapy, tooth #19

Apical
Chronic Apical Abscess, tooth #19 with cutaneous sinus tract

Treatment Plan
Recommended
Emergency: None
Definitive: Non-surgical root canal treatment (NSRCT) of tooth #19; informed consent obtained

Alternative
Extraction of tooth #19

Restorative
Core build-up and crown placement

Prognosis

Favorable	Questionable	Unfavorable
X		

Clinical Procedures: Treatment Record
First visit (Day 1): Vital signs were as follows: BP 115/60 mmHg; pulse 90 BPM. Pt was asymptomatic (ASX). Chief complaint was taken, medical history and dental history were reviewed (RMHX), the clinical evaluation, diagnosis, treatment options, and treatment (Tx) plan were discussed with Pt. PA and bitewing radiographs were taken. Tooth #19 showed no percussion, no palpation, mobility WNL, and probing less than 3 mm. The Tx options were reviewed with the Pt and his guardians including tooth saving through NSRCT versus tooth extraction. The Pt's legal guardians were informed about potential complications that might

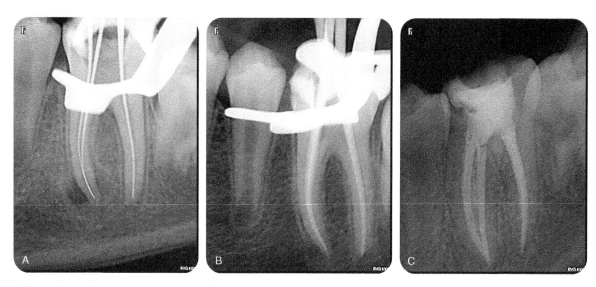

Figure 14.3 Periapical radiographs taken for working-length determination (A), master cone fit (B), and obturation (C).

occur during and after the procedures. NSRCT was chosen and informed consent was obtained. The Pt was scheduled for Tx at the end of the month.

Second visit (Day 29): RMHX. BP 112/51 mmHg, pulse 85 BPM. Pt was ASX. Local anesthesia; 3.6 mL of 2% Lidocaine (lido) with 1:100,000 epinephrine (epi) were administered for inferior alveolar nerve block (IANB) and long buccal nerve block on the left side. Single tooth (tooth #19) rubber dam isolation (RDI) was performed. Access cavity was done through the resin modified glass ionomer (RMGI) to warrant four-walled access cavity. Four canal orifices were detected (Mesiobuccal [MB], mesiolingual [ML], distobuccal [DB], and distolingual [DL] canals). Copious irrigation with saline was performed to flush the remaining non-setting Ca(OH)$_2$. Crown-down technique was performed. Coronal pre-flaring of the canals was done with ProFile® instrument size #40, .06 taper (Dentsply Sirona, Ballaigues, Switzerland). Irrigation with 6% sodium hypochlorite (NaOCl) was performed. The estimated working length (WL) was established with an electronic apex locator and adjusted for correct WL radiographically (Figure 14.3A). Shaping the canals was completed with K3™ rotary instrument size #35, .06 taper (SybronEndo, Orange, CA, USA) in the middle third, and size #30, .06 taper followed by size #35 .06 taper to the WL. The canals were further disinfected with 6% NaOCl and 17% Ethylenediaminetetraacetic acid (EDTA). The canals were then dried with paper points and filled

with non-setting Ca(OH)$_2$ by using a Lentulo® Spiral Filler (Dentsply Sirona, Ballaigues, Switzerland). The access opening was restored with RMGI. Postoperative instructions (POI) were given.

Third visit (6 months): RMHX. BP 124/66 mmHg, pulse 80 BPM. Pt was ASX. The extra-oral opening appeared to be healing with slight dimpling of the skin (Figure 14.4). Local anesthesia of 3.6 mL of 2% lido with 1:100,000 epi for IANB was administered. RDI was performed. Access preparation was performed. Non-setting Ca(OH)$_2$ was almost gone. After a rinse with NaOCl, WL was checked. After recapitulation, a final passive ultrasonic rinse was administered: 6% NaOCl, 17% EDTA, saline and then 2% chlorhexidine. Canals were dried with paper points. Cold lateral compaction technique was performed. AH Plus® Root

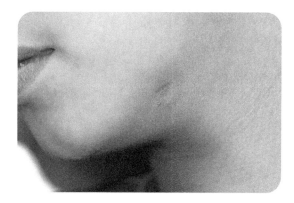

Figure 14.4 Extraoral image showing the sinus tract was healed with slight dimpling.

Canal Sealer (Dentsply Sirona, Konstanz, Germany) was applied. Master cones sizes #35, .06 taper were fit in the four canals (Figure 14.3B). Finger spreader size #30, .02 taper was used for compaction. Accessory cones were placed sequentially untill the canals were fully obturated (Figure 14.3C). Pulp chamber was cleaned with alcohol-moistened cotton pellet. Access cavity was closed with Cavit™ (3M, Two Harbors, MN, USA) and RMGI. Occlusion was checked (light contact with the opposing teeth). The Pt was scheduled for follow-up, and POI were given.

Working length, apical size, and obturation technique

Canal	Working Length	Apical Size, Taper	Obturation Materials and Techniques
MB	19.0 mm	35, .06	GP and AH Plus® Sealer, Cold lateral compaction
ML	19.0 mm	35, .06	GP and AH Plus® Sealer, Cold lateral compaction
DB	20.0 mm	35, .06	GP and AH Plus® Sealer, Cold lateral compaction
DL	20.0 mm	35, .06	GP and AH Plus® Sealer, Cold lateral compaction

Postoperative Evaluation

Fourth visit (3-month follow-up): The Pt was ASX and comfortable. Clinical examination revealed no signs of apical infection; the tooth was non-tender to percussion and there was no apical erythema, tenderness, or discharge. Radiographic examination showed considerable osseous healing around the M root except the apical area (Figure 14.5A).

The Pt failed to attend the six months postoperative evaluation.

Fifth visit (8-month follow-up): The Pt was ASX and comfortable. PA radiograph showed partial resolution of the periapical radiolucency (PARL) (Figure 14.5B).

Sixth visit (1-year follow-up): The Pt was ASX and comfortable. PA radiograph showed more resolution of the PARL. The RMGI was replaced with composite filling (Filtek™ Bulk Fill, 3M ESPE, Two Harbors, MN, USA) (Figure 14.5C).

Seventh visit (14-month follow-up): The Pt was ASX and comfortable. Adequate healing of the PA area with radiographic signs of reactive ostitis and traceable lamina dura was noted (Figure 14.5D).

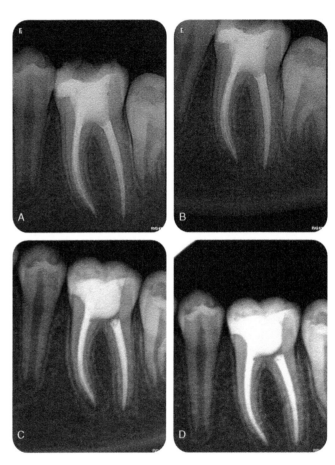

Figure 14.5 Recall radiographs after 3 months (A), 8 months (B), 12 months (C), and 14 months (D) intervals.

Self-Study Questions

A. What are the stages required to reach an endodontic diagnosis?

B. How is an odontogenic sinus tract formed, and what are the possible causes?

C. How do you manage a cutaneous sinus tract of odontogenic origin?

D. Why is "postoperative evaluation" imperative after endodontic treatment?

E. How do you determine the success of non-surgical root canal treatment?

Answers to Self-Study Questions

A. Since diagnosis is the first step in the care and management of any patient in endodontics, a systematic approach is necessary in order to provide proper treatment to manage the patient's complaint. The following stages are required to make an endodontic diagnosis (Berman & Rotstein 2015):

- Listening to the patient's presenting complaint and asking him about the symptoms and history of that complaint.
- Taking appropriate medical and dental histories.
- Examining the patient extra-orally as well as intra-orally.
- Performing and interpreting objective clinical and radiographic tests.
- Correlating the objective findings with the subjective information.

B. The major causative role of microbes in the pathogenesis of pulp and periapical diseases has been established (Kakehashi, Stanley & Fitzgerald 1965). Periapical diseases of endodontic origin are generated by an inflammatory reaction to pulpal necrosis and infection to prevent the spread of infection into periapical tissues. This reaction might result in a chronic inflammatory environment at the apical area which induces bone resorption. If the reaction is sustained, a sinus tract might form and drain intra-orally through the buccal or lingual/palatal cortices; occasionally the sinus tract might drain extra-orally into the skin (Ørstavik & Pitt Ford 2008). Cutaneous draining sinus can be caused by many diseases, such as suppurative apical periodontitis, osteomyelitis, an infected cyst, salivary gland infection, congenital anomalies, deep mycotic infection, foreign-body reaction, malignancy, and granulomatous disorders (Johnson, Remeikis & Van Cura 1999).

C. A cutaneous sinus tract of odontogenic origin is often treated improperly because of its relatively infrequent occurrence. Adequately performed non-surgical root canal treatment (NSRCT) is often an effective approach to manage a cutaneous sinus

tract of endodontic origin. The success of NSRCT depends mainly on the eradication of microbes from the root canal system by effective chemomechanical debridement. Canal shaping is performed to facilitate effective irrigation, disinfection, and obturation. Irrigants are used to flush out debris, dissolve organic and inorganic tissues, and eradicate microbes and their toxins. In infected teeth with chronic apical abscess, all debridement procedures followed by a quality obturation of the root canal should be performed close to the radiographic apex in order to regain healthy periapical tissues (Chugal, Clive & Spångberg 2003). Although the presence of apical periodontitis reduces the success rate of NSRCT, the treatment prognosis would be favorable when it is effectively performed under optimal conditions. It has been shown that cases with cutaneous sinus tracts of odontogenic origin adequately heal once the offending tooth is endodontically treated, and complete healing with a visible scar might occur on the skin area of the sinus tract (Soares *et al.* 2007). Delayed diagnosis or inadequate treatment of pulpal diseases might lead to unwanted complications such as sinus tract formation. Therefore, adequate debridement of the root canal system is essential to achieve healing of periapical inflammation and resolution of the draining sinus.

D. Regular recall is essential to evaluate treatment success, side effects, and the patient's overall progress, as well as to identify any necessary intervention that has been overlooked. It also allows the clinician to address any issues or complications following treatment.

E. Treatment outcome is evaluated by using clinical and radiographic measures. Clinical success criteria include normal mobility and function along with absence of signs and symptoms of infection including discomfort, pain, tenderness to percussion, swelling, sinus tract, periodontal pocket, sinusitis, and paresthesia. On the other hand, radiographic success criteria include normal periodontal ligament space, absence of furcal or apical radiolucency, and absence of bone and/or root resorption (Torabinejad & White 2015). Based on recall studies, endodontically treated teeth demonstrate significant successful outcome rates if the treatment is appropriately chosen and rendered (Setzer and Kim 2014).

References

Berman, L. & Rotstein, I. (2015) Diagnosis. In: *Cohen's Pathways of the Pulp* (eds. K. Hargreaves & L. Berman), 11th edn, pp. 2–24. St. Louis, MO: Elsevier.

Chugal, N. M., Clive, J. M. & Spångberg, L. S. (2003) Endodontic infection: Some biologic and treatment factors associated with outcome. *Oral Surgery, Oral Medicine, Oral Pathology, Oral Radiology, and Endodontics* **96**, 81–90.

Johnson, B. R., Remeikis, N. A. & Van Cura, J. E. (1999) Diagnosis and treatment of cutaneous facial sinus tracts of dental origin. *Journal of American Dental Association* **130**, 832–836.

Kakehashi, S., Stanley, H. R. & Fitzgerald, R. J. (1965) The effects of surgical exposures of dental pulps in germ-free and conventional laboratory rats. *Oral Surgery, Oral Medicine and Oral Pathology* **20**, 340–349.

Ørstavik, D. & Pitt Ford, T. (2008) Apical periodontitis: Microbial infection and host responses. In: *Essential Endodontology* (eds. D. Ørstavik & T. Pitt Ford), 2nd edn, pp. 2–9. Oxford: Blackwell.

Setzer, F. C. & Kim, S. (2014) Comparison of long-term survival of implants and endodontically treated teeth. *Journal of Dental Research* **93**, 19–26.

Soares, J. A., de Carvalho, F. B., Pappen, F. G. *et al.* (2007) Conservative treatment of patients with periapical lesions associated with extraoral sinus tracts. *Australian Endodontic Journal* **33**, 131–135.

Torabinejad, M. & White, S. (2015) Evaluation of endodontic outcomes. In: *Endodontics: Principles and Practice* (eds. M. Torabinejad, R. Walton & A. Fouad), 5th edn, pp. 397–411. St. Louis, MO: Elsevier.

15

Non-surgical Root Canal Treatment Case IX: Maxillary Molar / Difficult Anatomy (Dilacerated Molar Case Management)

Priya S. Chand and Jeffrey Albert

LEARNING OBJECTIVES
- To understand the diagnosis of this case according to the American Association of Endodontists (AAE) diagnostic terminology.
- To understand the complexity of this case according to the AAE Endodontic Case Difficulty Assessment form.
- To understand the management of dilacerated cases.

	Molars			Premolars		Canine	Incisors				Canine	Premolars		Molars		
						Maxillary arch										
Universal tooth designation system	1	2	3	4	5	6	7	8	9	10	11	12	13	14	15	16
International standards organization designation system	18	17	16	15	14	13	12	11	21	22	23	24	25	26	27	28
Palmer method	8⌋	7⌋	6⌋	5⌋	4⌋	3⌋	2⌋	1⌋	⌊1	⌊2	⌊3	⌊4	⌊5	⌊6	⌊7	⌊8
Palmer method	8⌉	7⌉	6⌉	5⌉	4⌉	3⌉	2⌉	1⌉	⌈1	⌈2	⌈3	⌈4	⌈5	⌈6	⌈7	⌈8
International standards organization designation system	48	47	46	45	44	43	42	41	31	32	33	34	35	36	37	38
Universal tooth designation system	32	31	30	29	28	27	26	25	24	23	22	21	20	19	18	17
						Mandibular arch										
		Right									**Left**					

Clinical Cases in Endodontics, First Edition. Edited by Takashi Komabayashi.
© 2018 John Wiley & Sons, Inc. Published 2018 by John Wiley & Sons, Inc.

Chief Complaint

"I have severe pain to cold on my upper left tooth. It hurts all of the time."

Medical History

The patient (Pt) was a 57-year-old Caucasian male. Blood pressure (BP) was 126/77 mmHg, pulse 64 beats per minute (BPM), respiratory rate (RR) 16 breaths per minute. Pt reported with a history of hypertension, arthritis, and no known drug allergies (NKDA). He managed his hypertension by regulating his diet and regular exercise. He also took metoprolol tartrate 100 mg daily for hypertension and ibuprofen 400 mg as needed for arthritic discomfort. The Pt denied respiratory, hematological, gastrointestinal, nervous system, or genitourinary disorders.

The Pt was American Society of Anesthiesiologists Physical Status Scale (ASA) Class II. There were no contraindications to routine dental treatment (Tx).

Dental History

The Pt was referred by his dentist for root canal treatment (RCT) on tooth #15. Three days prior, the dentist had placed a temporary (temp) bridge on abutments on teeth #12, #13, and #15 with pontic on tooth #14. Following the placement, the Pt had been experiencing severe, spontaneous, and cold drink pain in the upper left posterior quadrant. He reported that the teeth were asymptomatic prior to placing the temp bridge. The new bridge was being fabricated to replace an older faulty bridge that had recurrent decay on abutment on tooth #15. Tooth #14 was extracted over fifteen years ago. The Pt went for routine periodontal maintenance and yearly dental examinations. He had several crowns and dental restorations throughout the mouth.

Clinical Evaluation (Diagnostic Procedures)
Examinations
Extra-oral Examination (EOE)

The face was bilaterally symmetrical. Lymph nodes were not tender or enlarged. The oral cancer screening was negative.

Intra-oral Examination (IOE)

Teeth #12, #13, and #15 presented as abutments with a temp bridge. Tooth #14 was not present and a temp pontic was contacting the gingiva. The temp bridge had overhanging margins on all three teeth. Underneath the bridge, tooth #15 exhibited a mesio-occlusal (MO)

composite build-up with good marginal integrity. Teeth #12 and #13 did not have any restorations or caries present. Periodontal probings for teeth #12, #13, and #15 were 1–3 mm circumferentially. The temp bridge was removed and an endodontic examination was performed for teeth #12, #13, #15, and #19.

Diagnostic Tests

Tooth	#12	#13	#15	#19
Percussion	WNL	WNL	+	WNL
Palpation	WNL	WNL	WNL	WNL
Cold	WNL	WNL	L	WNL
EPT	+	+	+	+
Bite	WNL	WNL	+	WNL

EPT: Electric pulp test; WNL: within normal limits; L: Lingering; +: Positive response to percussion, EPT, or bite.

Radiographic Findings

One digital periapical radiograph (PAX) was taken (Figure 15.1). Normal trabecular pattern of bone was observed. The PAX showed teeth #13, #15, and part of tooth #12. Periodontal bone evaluation indicated mild bone loss. Tooth #15 revealed a radiopaque coronal restoration with an underlying more radiopaque restoration extending close to the pulp chamber. The pulp chamber appeared to be receded and the root canals were not easily visible. The mesiobuccal (MB) and distobuccal (DB) roots were dilacerated. The MB root displayed a sharp, almost 90° distal (D) curve in the middle third of the root. The DB root sharply curved to the D. The DB and palatal (P) root apices showed a thickened lamina dura, while the apical extent of the MB root was difficult to distinguish on the PAX. Tooth #14 was absent, with a radiopaque restoration attached to teeth #13 and #15. Tooth #13 showed a radiopaque

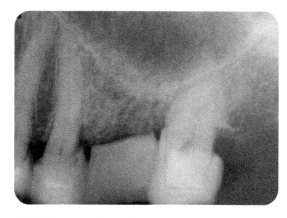

Figure 15.1 Preoperative radiograph.

coronal restoration, a receded pulp chamber, and an intact lamina dura apically. Tooth #12 was partially shown with a radiopaque coronal restoration and an intact lamina dura. Radiopacities were observed in the maxillary sinus apical to tooth #15.

Pretreatment Diagnosis
Pulpal
Symptomatic Irreversible Pulpitis, tooth #15

Apical
Symptomatic Apical Periodontitis, tooth #15

Treatment Plan
Recommended
Emergency: N/A
Definitive: Non-surgical root canal treatment

Alternative
Extraction and replacement prosthesis or no treatment with potential consequences

Restorative
Chamber retained core and cuspal coverage: Tx planned as a bridge abutment

Prognosis

Favorable	Questionable	Unfavorable
X		

Clinical Procedures: Treatment Record

First visit (Day 1): Options were presented to the Pt with both pros and cons of Tx. The Pt opted and consented for RCT on tooth #15. The temp bridge was removed prior to testing the teeth. 20% benzocaine topical anesthetic was placed and 68 mg of lidocaine (lido) with 0.034 mg epinephrine (epi) was administered by infiltration injection at the base of the buccal (B) vestibule, apical to tooth #15. A palatal infiltration injection was given. The rubber dam (RD) was placed on tooth #15 and an access cavity was prepared with a #2 carbide round bur. Examination of the pulp chamber with the surgical operating microscope revealed a heavily bleeding pulp with several pulp stones. The pulp stones were removed with ultrasonic vibration and an endodontic explorer. The MB and P canals were located, but the calcified DB and MB2 canals were not visualized with the microscope on the pulpal floor. An LN™ bur (Dentsply Sirona, Tulsa, OK, USA) was used to remove the calcified tissue over the DB canal and trough

the area of the MB2 canal. The DB canal was located 2 mm apical to the pulpal floor in the DB root. The MB2 canal could not be located. Gates-Glidden burs #2 and #3 were used to flare the coronal third of the root canals. Heavy canal calcifications were encountered in the MB and DB canals. After an hour of attempting to negotiate the three canals, the Pt showed signs of tiring. Working lengths (WL) were determined by the electronic apex locator (EAL) for the MB, DB, and P canals. The DB and P canals were instrumented to a size #25 K-file. The highly curved and calcified MB canal could only be cleaned and shaped to a size #15 K-file, needing to continually recapitulate to smaller files in order to maintain a clear canal path to the apex. The canals were irrigated with 10 ml of 5.25% sodium hypochlorite (NaOCl), 8 ml of 17% ethylenediaminetetraacetic acid (EDTA), and RC-Prep® (Premier Dental Products, Morristown, PA, USA) was used for file lubrication. Paper points were used to dry the canals and calcium hydroxide (Ca(OH)$_2$) paste was placed with a size #10 K-file to working length in all three canals. A dry cotton pellet was placed into the pulp chamber. The access cavity was sealed with Cavit™ G (3M, Two Harbors, MN, USA) and the temp bridge was cemented with Temp-Bond™ (Kerr, Romulus, MI, USA). The occlusion was verified with an articulating paper. The Pt felt well at dismissal and was instructed to take 600 mg ibuprofen every 6 hours as needed for discomfort. The Pt was scheduled to continue treatment in one week.

Second visit (Day 8): BP 122/72 mmHg, pulse 66 BPM. The Pt was asymptomatic (ASX). 20% benzocaine topical anesthetic was placed and 34 mg of lido with 0.017 mg epi was administered by infiltration injection at the base of the B vestibule, apical to tooth #15. A palatal infiltration injection was given. The temp bridge was removed and RCT on tooth #15 was continued under RD isolation. After tooth # 15 was re-accessed, WLs were confirmed by the EAL. Continued troughing in the area of the MB2 canal produced a stick with the endodontic explorer. The MB2 canal was calcified and curved. After 45 minutes of Tx, the MB and MB2 canals could only be negotiated to WL with a size #20 K-file. The MB and MB2 canals required additional flaring of the coronal third and continual recapitulation to smaller files in order to maintain a clear canal path to the apex. The DB and P canals were both cleaned and shaped to WL with a Vortex Blue® Nickel Titanium (NiTi) rotary files (Dentsply Sirona, Johnson City, TN, USA), size #30, .04 taper using a crown-down technique. Prior to using the rotary files a #25 K-file was used to verify the WLs with the EAL. The canals were irrigated with 10 ml of 5.25% NaOCl, 6 ml of

17% EDTA, and RC-Prep® was used for file lubrication. A final irrigation of 3 ml of 2% chlorhexidine (CHX) was performed. The Pt was tiring and a decision was made to complete the DB and P canals. Paper points were used to dry the canals and a cone fit PAX (Figure 15.2) was taken. (Note the file placed in the MB canal to confirm the working length). The radiograph showed a radiolucent area extending from the inferior border of the maxillary sinus to the coronal third of the root of tooth #13. The tooth was ASX and tested WNL to the cold test at the initial appointment. The periodontal probings were confirmed for teeth #12, #13, and #15 at 1–3mm circumferentially. The general dentist was notified and advised to have an oral surgeon review the radiograph and evaluate the Pt prior to placing the bridge. Obturation of the DB and P canals was completed by warm vertical compaction, using AH Plus® Root Canal Sealer (Dentsply Sirona, Konstanz, Germany) to coat the gutta-percha (GP) cones and canal walls. A heat source and pluggers were used to heat and compact the GP. The remaining canal space was backfilled with warm GP to the level of the canal orifices. Ca(OH)$_2$ paste was placed with a size #10 K-file to working length in the MB and MB2 canals. A dry cotton pellet was placed in the pulp chamber. The access cavity was sealed with Cavit™ G and the temp bridge was cemented with Temp-Bond™. The occlusion was verified with an articulating paper. The Pt felt well at dismissal and postoperative instructions (POI) were reviewed. A one-week completion appointment for the MB and MB2 canals was scheduled.

Third visit (Day 14): BP 118/74 mmHg, pulse 62 BPM. The Pt was ASX. Tooth #13 tested WNL to the cold test. 20% benzocaine topical anesthetic was placed and 34 mg of lido with 0.017 mg epi was administered by infiltration injection at the base of B vestibule, apical to tooth #15. A palatal infiltration injection was given. The

temp bridge was removed and RCT of tooth #15 was completed under rubber dam isolation (RDI). Tooth #15 was re-accessed, and WLs for the MB and MB2 canals were confirmed by the EAL. The canals were instrumented to WL to a #25 K-file. The MB and MB2 canals were cleaned and shaped with Vortex Blue® Nickel Titanium (NiTi) rotary files (Dentsply Sirona, Johnson City, TN, USA) using a crown-down technique to a size #30, .04 taper and size #25, .04 taper, respectively. The canals were irrigated with 6 ml of 5.25% NaOCl, 4 ml of 17% EDTA, and RC-Prep® was used for file lubrication. A final irrigation of 3 ml of 2% CHX was performed. Paper points were used to dry the canals and a cone fit radiograph was taken. The MB and MB2 canals joined in the apical 1–2 mm of the M root. Obturation of the canals were completed by warm vertical compaction using the same protocol as described in the previous visit. The pulp chamber was cleaned with an alcohol cotton pellet. A dry cotton pellet was placed in the pulp chamber and the access cavity was sealed with Cavit™ G. The temp bridge was cemented with Temp-Bond™ and the occlusion was verified with articulating paper. Two final digital PAX (Figures 15.3 and 15.4) were taken showing well obturated canals to within 0.5 mm of the

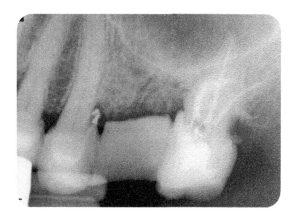

Figure 15.3 Final fill radiograph 1.

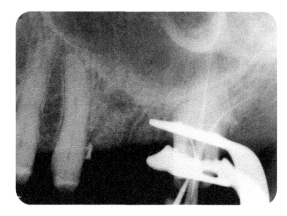

Figure 15.2 Master cone gutta-percha fit radiograph.

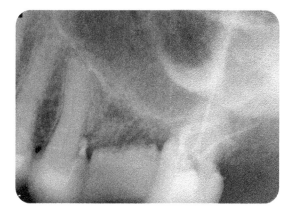

Figure 15.4 Final fill radiograph 2.

radiographic apices. The MB1 and MB2 canals joined in the apical 1–2 mm. The radiolucency mentioned during the previous visit, cone fit PAX, was not as evident in the two final PAX. The dentist was advised of the radiolucent area in close proximity to the sinus. The Pt felt well at dismissal and POI were reviewed. The Pt scheduled an appointment to return to his dentist in the next two weeks to proceed with the fabrication of the new bridge for teeth #12 to #15.

Working length, apical size, and obturation technique

Canal	Working Length	Apical Size, Taper	Obturating Materials and Technique
MB	17.0 mm	30, .04	GP and AH Plus® sealer, Warm vertical compaction
MB2	18.0 mm	25, .04	GP and AH Plus® sealer, Warm vertical compaction
DB	19.0 mm	30, .04	GP and AH Plus® sealer, Warm vertical compaction
P	19.5 mm	30, .04	GP and AH Plus® sealer, Warm vertical compaction

Postoperative Evaluation

Fourth visit (1-year follow-up): Clinical examination; BP 128/83 mmHg; pulse 69 BPM. There were no changes in the medical Hx. EOE showed bilateral symmetry of the face. Lymph nodes were not tender or enlarged. IOE was unremarkable. The oral cancer screening was negative.

The Pt was ASX. Teeth #12, #13, and #15 were WNL for percussion, palpation, and bite. Teeth #12 and #13 were WNL to the cold test. The dental Hx included a new bridge on abutment teeth #12, #13, and #15 with pontic tooth #14. Periodontal probings were 2–3 mm circumferentially for teeth #12 to #15. The gingiva appeared pink and healthy. The occlusion was WNL, verified with articulating paper. The bridge margins appeared to be well sealed as inspected with the dental explorer.

Radiographic examination: two digital PAX were taken. PAX (Figure 15.5) showed an intact lamina dura apically on the DB root of tooth #15. The root canals were well obturated to within 0.5 mm of the radiographic apices. The MB1 and MB2 canals joined in the apical 1–2 mm of the root. PAX (Figure 15.6) revealed a second angle of tooth #15 and the DB root apex was not shown. The radiolucent area in the proximity of the sinus was not clearly visible. The Pt did not see an oral surgeon as advised.

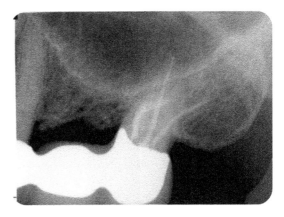

Figure 15.5 One-year recall radiograph 1.

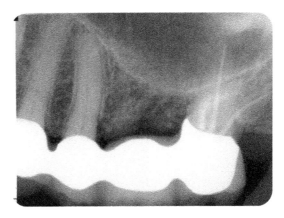

Figure 15.6 One-year recall radiograph 2.

Self-Study Questions

A. How do you define dilacerations and what is the prevalence of dilacerated roots in endodontics?

B. What are the technical considerations for management of dilacerated root canals?

C. What are the current advancements in endodontic approaches to complex clinical cases?

D. What are the risks associated with managing a dilacerated root canal?

E. What are the factors that can affect the prognosis for this case?

Answers to Self-Study Questions

A. The term dilaceration, first used by Tomes in 1848, refers to a sharp bend or curve in the root or crown of a formed tooth. It can also be defined as a deviation or bend in the linear relationship of a crown to its root. According to some authors (Hamasha, Al-Khateeb & Darwazeh 2002), a tooth is considered to have a dilaceration toward the mesial or distal direction if there is a 90° angle or greater curve along the axis of the tooth or root. In contrast, others define dilaceration as a deviation from the normal axis of the tooth, 20° or more in the apical part of the root (Chohayeb 1983).

Dilaceration has been observed in both permanent and deciduous dentitions, but the incidence in the latter is very low (Bimstein 1978; Neville *et al.* 2002). Some researchers have reported that the prevalence is greater in posterior teeth and in the maxilla. There are fewer occurrences among anterior teeth and in the mandible. Furthermore, bilaterally occurring dilacerations might be seen in many patients (Ng *et al.* 2008), but bilateral dilaceration in both the maxilla and mandible of the same person is rarely found. There is no sex predilection for dilacerations of teeth.

B. First, it is important to recognize the complexity of the case and to formulate a customized treatment plan for the management of curved canals. A step by step guide used to treat curved canals and reduce incidence of procedural errors is outlined below (Sakkir *et al.* 2014)

Access: In order to provide the most direct access to the apical foramen, enough tooth structure must be removed to allow the endodontic instruments to move freely within the coronal cavity. However, an important observation outlined by Luebke (Ingle *et al.* 2002) states that an entire access cavity wall does not need to be extended in the event that instrument impingement occurs as a result of a dilacerated root. (Ingle *et al.* 2002) In extending only the portion of the wall needed to free the instrument, a cloverleaf appearance is created as the outline form. Luebke has termed this a "shamrock preparation." (Ingle *et al.* 2002) This is a modified

outline form to accommodate the instrument, unrestrained in severely curved canals.

Decreasing the restoring force caused by a straight file bending against the curved dentine surface can be done by the following:
1. Precurving the file: A precurved file traverses the curve better than a straight file. Precurving is performed in two ways:
   - Placing a gradual curve for the entire length of the file
   - Placing a sharp curve of nearly 45° near the apical end of the instrument
2. Use of smaller number files: Smaller files have a better ability to follow the canal curvature due to their flexibility. It is recommended that the smaller sized files negotiate the canal loosely prior to proceeding to the subsequent file size.
3. Use of intermediate file sizes: These files allow for an easier transition of instrument sizes resulting in smoother cutting in curved canals. Cutting 1 mm from the apex of a size #15 file converts it to a size #17 file as there is an increase of 0.02 mm of diameter per 1 mm of length.
4. Use of flexible files (nickel-titanium files, Flex-R® files): These files help in maintaining the shape of the curved canal and avoid procedural errors like ledging, elbowing, or zipping of the root canal.

Decreasing the length of actively cutting files is achieved by: Anti-curvature filing or modifying the cutting edges of the instrument by dulling the flute on the outer surface of the apical third and inner portion of the middle third. This can be performed using a diamond file. Another way to accomplish this is by changing the canal preparation techniques, i.e., use of coronal pre-flaring and crown-down technique.

C. According to Kishen *et al.* (2016), contemporary endodontics has seen unprecedented advancement in technology and materials, impacting all aspects of the specialty.
1. Endodontic imaging: The advent of cone beam computed tomography (CBCT) has resulted in widespread adoption of this technology for 3-D

image capture and processing. CBCT greatly enhances diagnostic ability in circumstances when 2-D conventional radiographic interpretation has limitations.

2. Root canal preparation: Engine-driven instrumentation with nickel-titanium (NiTi alloy) continues to be used more frequently by endodontists compared to hand instruments. Improved rotary instruments are constantly being introduced with the invention of more flexible alloys. This increased flexibility promises better canal negotiation and an extended fatigue life. Reciprocating motion techniques can reduce the number of instruments used per patient. In addition, the greatly improved NiTi files are designed to instrument a larger area of the canal wall and to decrease the need for coronal flaring.

3. Root canal disinfection: Current advances in endodontic disinfection are geared towards improving fluid dynamics during root canal irrigation. This is accomplished by improving bubble dynamics, activating intensified cavitational bubbles, and utilizing more effective antimicrobials. One example is developing irrigants that demonstrate improved antibiofilm effects over sodium hypochlorite.

4. Root canal filling: In recent years, new concepts have evolved that can improve and facilitate root-filling procedures. One example is to use a calcium silicate cement-based sealer. These sealers are initially flowable and express bioactive properties, i.e., they promote Ca/P precipitation in a wet environment. The interface that forms between the sealer and the root canal wall is calcium phosphate and, thus, mimics nature. However, a core material, gutta-percha is still necessary.

These advances are aimed towards improving contemporary Endodontics and enhancing state of the art treatment approaches needed to successfully complete complex cases.

D. According to Hamasha *et al.* (2002), dilacerated canals can pose significant challenges to clinicians.

Failures in treating dilacerated root canal cases result from an inability to maintain the natural anatomic root canal curvature. This may lead to the formation of ledges, apical transportation, zipping, perforation, or instrument breakage. In order to avoid these mishaps, the basic principles of endodontic therapy must be followed. These include good preoperative radiographs, straight-line access to the apical foramen, precurving the endodontic hand instruments, recapitulation, copious irrigation, and the use of flexible NiTi instruments.

E. Prognosis of this case as defined by the American Association of Endodontic Terminology would be categorized as favorable. However, prognosis depends on several factors including diagnosis. According to Sjogren *et al.* (1990), success rates are: vital teeth: 96% success rate – no microorganisms; PN (necrosis)–PL (lesion): 86%; PN–PL with overfill less than 2 mm: 76%; PN–PL with underfill more than 2 mm: 68%.

In a study by Ng *et al.* (2008), four conditions were found to significantly improve the outcome of primary root canal treatment. These conditions include the preoperative absence of a periapical radiolucency, a root filling with no voids present, the obturation extending within 2 mm of the radiographic apex, and a satisfactory coronal restoration. Consequently, the goals of successful root canal treatment are to maintain access to the apical anatomy during chemomechanical debridement, to obturate the canal with densely compacted material to the apical terminus without extrusion into the apical tissues, and to prevent reinfection with a good quality coronal restoration. In the Toronto study (de Chevigny *et al.* 2008), the outcome of root canal treatment was assessed after 4–6 years. In teeth with radiolucencies, intra-operative complications (OR, 2.27; CI, 1.05–4.89; healed: absent, 84%; present, 69%) and root-filling technique (OR, 1.89; CI, 1.01–3.53; healed: lateral, 77%; vertical, 87%) were additional outcome predictors. A better outcome was reported for teeth without radiolucencies, with single roots, and without mid-treatment complications.

References

Bimstein, E. (1978) Root dilaceration and stunting in two unerupted primary incisors. *ASDC Journal of Dentistry for Children* **45**, 223–225.

Chohayeb, A. A. (1983) Dilaceration of permanent upper lateral incisors: Frequency, direction, and endodontic treatment implications. *Oral Surgery, Oral Medicine, and Oral Pathology* **55**, 519–520.

de Chevigny, C., Dao, T. T., Basrani, B. R. *et al.* (2008) Treatment outcome in endodontics: The Toronto study – Phase 4: Initial treatment. *Journal of Endodontics* **34** 258–263.

Hamasha, A. A., Al-Khateeb, T. & Darwazeh, A. (2002) Prevalence of dilaceration in Jordanian adults. *International Endodontic Journal* **35**, 910–912.

Ingle J.I, Himel, V.B., Hawrish, C.E. *et al.* (2002) Endodontic cavity preparation. In: *Endodontics* (eds. J.I. Ingle & L.K. Bakland), 5th edn, pp. 409, 465. London: B.C. Decker, Inc.

Kishen, A., Peters, O. A., Zehnder, M. *et al.* (2016) Advances in endodontics: Potential applications in clinical practice. *Journal of Conservative Dentistry* **19**, 199–206.

Neville, B. W., Damm, D. D., Allen, C. M. *et al.* (2002) Oral and maxillofacial pathology. In: *Oral and Maxillofacial Pathology* (eds. B. W. Neville, D. D. Damm, C. M. Allen *et al.*), 2nd edn, pp. 86–88. Philadelphia: W. B. Saunders.

Ng, Y. L., Mann, V., Rahbaran, S. *et al.* (2008) Outcome of primary root canal treatment: Systematic review of the literature – Part 2. Influence of clinical factors. *International Endodontic Journal* **41**, 6–31.

Sakkir, N., Thaha, K. A., Nair, M. J. *et al.* (2014) Management of dilacerated and S-shaped root canals – An endodontist's challenge. *Journal of Clinical and Diagnostic Research* **8**, ZD22–ZD24.

Sjogren, U., Hagglund, B., Sundqvist, G. *et al.* (1990) Factors affecting the long-term results of endodontic treatment. *Journal of Endodontics* **16**, 498–504.

Tomes, J. (1846–1848) A course of lectures on dental physiology and surgery (lectures I–XV). *American Journal of Dental Science* **7**, 1–68 & 121–134, **8**, 33–54, 120–147, & 313–350.

16

Non-Surgical Re-treatment Case I: Maxillary Anterior

Kana Chisaka-Miyara

LEARNING OBJECTIVES
- To understand the cause of failure of initial endodontic treatment.
- To determine the factor of pathosis by tracing the sinus tract with a gutta-percha point.
- To recognize when treatment requires two or more visits.
- To understand how to treat blocked or ledged canals.

	Molars			Premolars		Canine	Incisors				Canine	Premolars		Molars		
							Maxillary arch									
Universal tooth designation system	1	2	3	4	5	6	7	8	9	10	11	12	13	14	15	16
International standards organization designation system	18	17	16	15	14	13	12	11	21	22	23	24	25	26	27	28
Palmer method	8⌋	7⌋	6⌋	5⌋	4⌋	3⌋	2⌋	1⌋	⌊1	⌊2	⌊3	⌊4	⌊5	⌊6	⌊7	⌊8

	Molars			Premolars		Canine	Incisors				Canine	Premolars		Molars		
Palmer method	8⌉	7⌉	6⌉	5⌉	4⌉	3⌉	2⌉	1⌉	⌈1	⌈2	⌈3	⌈4	⌈5	⌈6	⌈7	⌈8
International standards organization designation system	48	47	46	45	44	43	42	41	31	32	33	34	35	36	37	38
Universal tooth designation system	32	31	30	29	28	27	26	25	24	23	22	21	20	19	18	17
							Mandibular arch									

Right	Left

Clinical Cases in Endodontics, First Edition. Edited by Takashi Komabayashi.
© 2018 John Wiley & Sons, Inc. Published 2018 by John Wiley & Sons, Inc.

Chief Complaint

"My gum near the upper front teeth on the right side is swelling."

Medical History

The patient (Pt) was a 42-year-old Asian male. Vital signs were as follows: blood pressure (BP) 120/80 mmHg. The Pt was taking medicine for hypertension, which was well-controlled.

Pt was American Society of Anesthesiologists Physical Status Scale (ASA) Class II.

Dental History

The Pt had caries on tooth #7 about twenty years ago and subsequent root canal treatment and restoration with composite resin by his general dentist. Six months ago, the Pt began experiencing acute pain on tooth #7, and then swelling. Incision for drainage was performed by his general dentist. Last month, the dentist referred him to see an endodontist for treatment because of the recurrence of sinus tract swelling.

Clinical Evaluation (Diagnostic Procedures)
Examinations
Extra-oral Examination (EOE)

Clinical examination revealed no lymphadenopathy of the submandibular and neck areas.

Perioral and extra-oral soft tissue appeared normal.

Intra-oral Examination (IOE)

A buccal (B) sinus tract was situated between teeth #7 and #8 (Figure 16.1). A B gum on tooth #8 formed the small fibrous tissue. The Pt's oral hygiene was acceptable. Periodontal depths of 2–3 mm were measured around the circumference of the tooth. The mesial (M) area was restored with a composite resin.

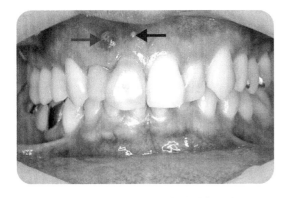

Figure 16.1 Intraoral photograph with draining sinus tract (red arrow) and a fibrous tissue (blue arrow).

Diagnostic Tests

Tooth	#6	#7	#8
Percussion	–	+	–
Palpation	–	+	–
CO$_2$ snow	+	N/A	N/A
EPT	+	N/A	N/A

EPT: Electric pulp test; +: Response to percussion or palpation, and normal response to CO$_2$ snow, or EPT; –: No response to percussion or palpation: N/A: Not applicable

Radiographic Findings

Tooth #7 showed radiolucent composite resin restoration at the M area. The root apex had 7 mm periradicular radiolucency with suboptimal root filling. Tooth #8 showed radiolucent composite resin restoration on the distal (D) area. The root canal filling reached 1 mm point from the radiographic apex. A gutta-percha (GP) point was inserted into the sinus tract to trace the source and the radiograph taken confirmed the tooth to which the tracing of the sinus tract led was tooth #7 (Figure 16.2 A, B).

Pretreatment Diagnosis
Pulpal

Previously Treated, tooth #7

Apical

Chronic Apical Abscess, tooth #7

Treatment Plan
Recommended

Emergency: None
Definitive: Re-treatment of tooth #7

Alternative

Root-end surgery of tooth #7 or extraction of tooth #7

Restorative

Permanent crown

Prognosis

Favorable	Questionable	Unfavorable
X		

Clinical Procedures: Treatment Record

First visit (Day 1): A periapical (PA) and an axial occlusal radiograph were taken with GP points from the B sinus tract located between teeth #7 and #8 (Figure 16.2 A, B).

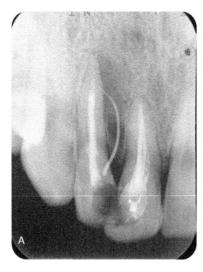
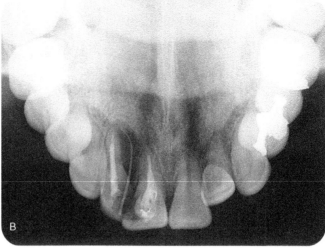

Figure 16.2 Pretreatment radiographs with gutta-percha point positioned in the sinus tract, pointing toward the tooth #7. A: Periapical radiograph. B: Axial occlusal radiograph.

The treatment (Tx) options were reviewed with the Pt including re-treatment (re-Tx) and apical surgery. The re-Tx of tooth #7 was recommended because of caries around the composite resin filling margin and the insufficient condensation and it was explained to the Pt that tooth #7 might have root fracture. The Pt agreed with this plan and informed consent was obtained.

Second visit (3 months): Diagnostic tests showed: Spontaneous pain (-), percussion pain (+), palpation (+), sinus tract (+). Anesthesia, 1.8 ml of 2% lidocaine (lido) with 1:100,000 epinephrine (epi) was administered. The tooth was isolated with a rubber dam (RD). Composite restoration and carious dentine were removed. Root filling material was removed with Gates-Glidden burs and the ultra-sonic tip under the dental operating microscope (OPMI® pico, Carl Zeiss, Oberkochen, Germany). The canal was instrumented short of the apex because the apical part was constricted. After antimicrobial medicament was placed, the tooth was sealed with a wet sponge and a temporary (temp) filling (Caviton® EX, GC Corporation, Tokyo, Japan).

Third visit (4 months): Diagnostic tests showed: Spontaneous pain (-), percussion pain (-), palpation (-), sinus tract (+). Anesthesia, consisting of 1.8 ml of 2% lidocaine (lido) with 1:100,000 epineferine (epi), was administered. The tooth was isolated with a RD. The patency was achieved, and the canal was prepared to the apical size #40 with hand instruments, K-files (Zipperer, Munich, Germany), and irrigated with 3% sodium hypochlorite (NaOCl; Dental Antiformin, Nippon

Shika Yakuhin, Yamaguchi, Japan). The working length (WL) was estimated using an electronic apex locator (Root ZX®II, J. Morita, Kyoto, Japan).

Fourth visit (6 months): Diagnostic tests showed: Spontaneous pain (–), percussion pain (-), palpation (–), sinus tract (+). Anesthesia, consisting of 1.8 ml of 2% lido with 1:100,000 epi, was administered. The tooth was isolated with a RD. The canal was irrigated with 14% Ethylenediaminetetraacetic acid (EDTA, Showa Yakuhin Kako, Tokyo, Japan) and 3% NaOCl. The canal was obturated by lateral (L) compaction of GP, using Canals®-N sealer (Showa Yakuhin Kako, Tokyo, Japan). A PA radiograph was taken (Figure 16.3).

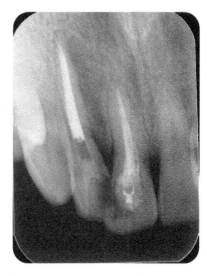

Figure 16.3 Post-treatment radiograph.

Working length, apical size, and obturation technique

Canal	Working Length	Apical Size, Taper	Obturation Materials and Techniques
Single	23.5 mm	40, .06	Gutta-percha, zinc oxide non-eugenol sealer, Lateral condensation

Postoperative Evaluation

Fifth visit (3-month follow-up): The PA radiograph (Figure 16.4) showed osseous healing in progress around the root apex. Tooth #7 was restored with the resin core (Clearfil™ DC Core Automix, Kuraray Noritake Dental, Nigata, Japan). The tooth was functional with no signs of swelling or sinus tract. The Pt was symptom-free. The radiograph indicated periradicular healing.

Sixth visit (6-month follow-up): Significant healing of the previous radiolucent area was noted on radiograph (Figure 16.5 A, B). The tooth was functional with no signs of swelling or sinus tract. The Pt was symptom-free. The tooth was restored with full crown.

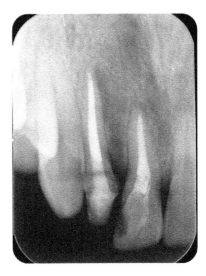

Figure 16.4 Three-month recall radiograph.

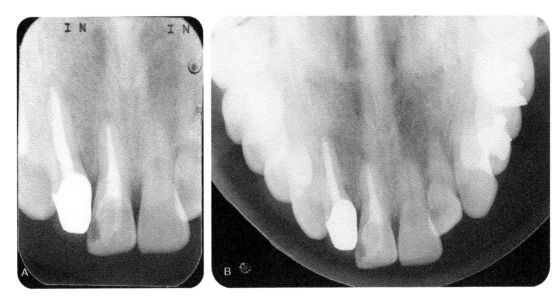

Figure 16.5 Six-month recall radiographs. A: Periapical radiograph. B: Axial occlusal radiograph.

Self-Study Questions

A. How are teeth with blocked and ledged canals treated?

B. Why is initial treatment sometimes a failure?

C. How is a tooth-caused sinus tract traced?

D. What are the important points in cases involving multiple visits?

E. For which cases are multiple visits recommended?

Answers to Self-Study Questions

A. A blocked canal contains residual pulp tissue. This debris is frequently infected, resulting in persistent disease, and must be removed if possible (Jafarzadeh & Abbott 2007). A ledge is a type of canal transportation that results in irregular shaping on the outside of the canal curvature. The ledge makes it difficult to detect the original canal. The best treatment for blocked and ledged canals is to prevent their occurrence. If the clinician is careful during instrumentation, the chances for blocked and ledged canals to develop are minimized (Roda & Gettleman 2011). Blocks and ledges may be detectible on radiographs as a root filling short of the ideal working length. However, short filling should not be performed in re-treatment (Farzaneh, Abitbol & Friedman 2004). When a block or ledge is encountered, the coronal portion of the canal should be enlarged to enhance tactile impression. Frequent irrigation should be performed to remove the debris that could block access. The obstacle should be gently probed with a pre-curved size #10 K-file to determine if there are any "sticky" spots that could be the entrance to a blocked canal. Frequent irrigation and use of a lubricant such as RC-Prep® enhances the ability to place a small file into the apical canal (Roda & Gettleman 2011). A K-file is useful for penetrating and enlarging root canals. When the negotiation with watch-winding motion results in some resistance, the clinician should continue to negotiate until further apical advancement is accomplished. Once apical working length is achieved, apical patency should be confirmed using an electric apex locator. If a sticky spot cannot be found, the clinician must consider the possible presence of a ledge. This technique is useful for ledged canals. After detecting the original canals, shaping is performed as usual.

B. The following are examples of reasons for failure of initial treatment:

Persistent or reintroduced intra-radicular microorganisms: When the root canal space and dentinal tubules are contaminated with microorganisms, and allowed to contact the periradicular tissues, apical periodontitis develops. Inadequate clean-ing, shaping, obturation, and final restoration of an endodontically diseased tooth can lead to posttreatment disease (Roda & Gettleman 2011). If initial endodontic treatment does not leave the canal space free of bacteria, if the obturation does not adequately entomb those that may remain (Siqueira & Rôças 2008), or if new microorganisms are allowed to re-enter the cleaned and sealed canal space, posttreatment disease can and usually does occur.

Extra-radicular infection: Bacterial cells can invade the periradicular tissues by spread of infection from the root canal space through contaminated periodontal pockets that communicate with the apical area, through extrusion of infected debris, or by use of infected endodontic instruments (Simon, Glick & Frank 1972).

Foreign body reaction: Persistent endodontic disease occurs in the absence of discernable microorganisms and has been attributed to the presence of foreign material in the periradicular area. Several materials have been associated with inflammatory responses (Roda & Gettleman 2011). Generally, filling material extrusion leads to a lower incidence of healing.

True cysts: The incidence of periapical cysts has been reported to be 15–42% of all periapical lesions (Roda & Gettleman 2011). It is hard to determine radiographically whether periapical radiolucency is a cyst or not (Bhaskar & Rappaport 1971).

C. The sinus tract is useful to detect the source of a given infection. The opening of the sinus tract may be located directly adjacent to or at a distant site from the infection (Roda & Gettleman 2011). Tracing the sinus tract will provide objectivity in diagnosing the location of the problem tooth. To trace the sinus tract, a size #25–#35 gutta-percha cone is threaded into the opening of the sinus tract. Although this may be slightly uncomfortable to the patient, the cone should be inserted until resistance is obtained. After a periapical radiograph is taken, the gutta-percha cone detects the location of the pathosis.

D. The canals are dressed with setting calcium hydroxide, and 3.5 mm of temporary filling is placed to decrease bacterial leakage.

E. The following are examples of cases warranting multiple visits:
- There is a clinical symptom such as pain, swelling, or sinus tract.

- The prognosis is difficult to predict and therapeutic effect must be evaluated.
- There is bleeding, discharge of pus, or exudate at the apex.
- Mechanical shaping isn't finished.

References

Bhaskar, S. N. & Rappaport, H. M. (1971) Histologic evaluation of endodontic procedures in dogs. *Oral Surgery, Oral Medicine, Oral Pathology* **31**, 526–535.

Farzaneh, M., Abitbol, S. & Friedman, S. (2004) Treatment outcome in endodontics: The Toronto Study. Phases I and II: Orthograde retreatment. *Journal of Endodontics* **30,** 627–633.

Jafarzadeh, H. & Abbott, P. V. (2007) Ledge formation: Review of a great challenge in endodontics. *Journal of Endodontics* **33**, 1155–1162.

Roda, R. S. & Gettleman, B. H. (2011) Nonsurgical retreatment. In: *Cohen's Pathways of the Pulp* (eds K. M. Hargreaves & S. Cohen), 10th edn, pp. 890–952. St. Louis, MO: Mosby.

Simon, J. H., Glick, D. H. & Frank, A. L. (1972) The relationship of endodontic-periodontic lesions. *Journal of Periodontology* **43**, 202–208.

Siqueira, J. F. Jr. & Rôças, I. N. (2008) Clinical implications and microbiology of bacterial persistence after treatment procedures. *Journal of Endodontics* **34**, 1291–1301.

17

Non-surgical Re-treatment Case II: Maxillary Premolar

Yoshio Yahata

LEARNING OBJECTIVES

- To understand the difference between root canal re-treatment and initial treatment.
- To appreciate the difficulty of root canal re-treatment.
- To understand the clinical success rate for re-treatment.
- To understand the methods and techniques of root canal re-treatment.

	Molars			Premolars		Canine	Incisors				Canine	Premolars		Molars		
							Maxillary arch									
Universal tooth designation system	1	2	3	4	5	6	7	8	9	10	11	12	13	14	15	16
International standards organization designation system	18	17	16	15	14	13	12	11	21	22	23	24	25	26	27	28
Palmer method	8⌋	7⌋	6⌋	5⌋	4⌋	3⌋	2⌋	1⌋	⌊1	⌊2	⌊3	⌊4	⌊5	⌊6	⌊7	⌊8
Palmer method	8⌉	7⌉	6⌉	5⌉	4⌉	3⌉	2⌉	1⌉	⌈1	⌈2	⌈3	⌈4	⌈5	⌈6	⌈7	⌈8
International standards organization designation system	48	47	46	45	44	43	42	41	31	32	33	34	35	36	37	38
Universal tooth designation system	32	31	30	29	28	27	26	25	24	23	22	21	20	19	18	17
							Mandibular arch									
	Right										**Left**					

Clinical Cases in Endodontics, First Edition. Edited by Takashi Komabayashi.
© 2018 John Wiley & Sons, Inc. Published 2018 by John Wiley & Sons, Inc.

Chief Complaint

"I have a long-term dull pain around the right upper molar and premolar area."

Medical History

The patient (Pt) was a 34-year-old male. He had no relevant medical history and was not taking any medications at the time of visit. His vital signs were as follows: blood pressure (BP) 132/87 mmHg; pulse 78 beats per minute (BPM) and regular. A complete review of systems did not reveal any significant findings and there were no contraindications to treatment.

The Pt was American Society of Anesthesiologists Physical Status Scale (ASA) Class I.

Dental History

Three years before presentation, the Pt experienced dull pain around his right upper posteriors. After visiting a dental office, root canal treatment (RCT) was performed on teeth #3 and #4, and tooth #5 was extracted. Following treatment (Tx), his discomfort reduced but slight pain remained. A referral dentist observed changes in his discomfort for two years under temporary (temp) restorations. However, during the follow-up, two months before presentation, he experienced dull pain around the same area. Although the dentist initiated RCT for tooth #3, the pain was not resolved and he was referred to the University hospital.

Clinical Evaluation (Diagnostic Procedures) Examinations
Extra-oral Examination (EOE)

The EOE did not reveal any significant findings, lymphadenopathy, or extra-oral swelling. There was no discomfort on opening or closing of the temporomandibular joint (TMJ), and no popping or clicking, or deviation to either side upon opening.

Intra-oral Examination (IOE)

The IOE revealed slight redness around the gingiva adjacent to teeth #3 and #4. These teeth had temp restorations (Figure 17.1).

Diagnostic Tests

Tooth	#2	#3	#4	#6
Percussion	–	+	+	–
Palpation	–	+	+	–
Cold	+	–	–	+
Probing depth	Within 3 mm	Within 3 mm	Within 3 mm	Within 3 mm

+: Response to pain on percussion or palpation and normal response to cold test; –: No response to percussion, palpation, or cold

Radiographic Findings

Periapical (PA) radiography (Figure 17.2) indicated that tooth #2 was free from decay and restorations, while tooth #3 indicated initiation of RCT with traces of root canal medication inside the root canals. Well-defined radiolucency of 1 mm diameter was associated with the apex of tooth #4. The root canal of this tooth had been previously insufficiently filled with material that was 3–4 mm short from the apex. A wide root canal suggested excessive removal of dentin by previous Tx. The remaining coronal tooth structure was insufficient. Tooth #5 was missing.

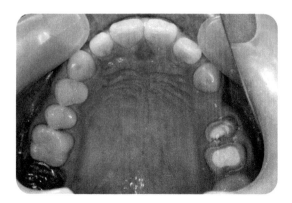

Figure 17.1 Intraoral photograph. Note: Root canal treatment has already been initiated as retreatment in teeth #3 and #4. In each tooth, access is sealed with Cavit™ temporary filling material.

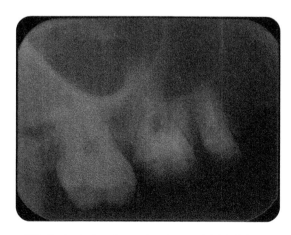

Figure 17.2 Periapical radiograph taken at initial visit.

Pretreatment Diagnosis
Pulpal
Previously Treated, tooth #4

Apical
Symptomatic Apical Periodontitis, tooth #4

Treatment Plan
Recommended
Emergency: None
Definitive: Non-surgical Re-treatment of tooth #4

Alternative
Extraction of tooth #4 or no treatment

Restorative
Core build-up and full crown coverage

Prognosis

Favorable	Questionable	Unfavorable
	X	

Clinical Procedures: Treatment Record

First visit (Day 1): Informed consent was obtained. Endodontic evaluation and the Tx plan were discussed with the Pt. Alternative Txs were also explained. For tooth #4, local anesthesia was administrated by infiltration of 1.8 ml of 2% XYLOCAINE® anesthetic with 1:80,000 epinephrine (epi) (Dentsply Sirona, Tokyo, Japan). The temporary restoration was removed and rubber dam isolation (RDI) was placed, followed by access and removal of the cement "core." After locating the canal orifice, the gutta-percha (GP) was removed using Gates–Glidden drills, hand and NiTi rotary files (EndoWave, J. Morita, Osaka, Japan) with the adjunctive use of eucalyptus oil (Eucaly soft plus®, Toyokagaku Kenkyusho, Tokyo, Japan). An operating microscope (Zeiss OPMI® pico, Carl Zeiss Meditec AG, Oberkochen, Germany) was used to verify the complete removal of previously filled GP. Working length (WL) was obtained as 13 mm using an electric apex locator (Root ZX®II, J. Morita, Kyoto, Japan). Cleaning and shaping was performed utilizing .02 taper stainless steel K-files. Irrigation with 5% sodium hypochlorite (NaOCl) using a 27-gauge needle was performed throughout the procedure. The canal was then dried with sterile paper points and medicated with calcium hydroxide (Ca(OH)$_2$; Calcipex® II, Nishika, Yamaguchi, Japan). Access was sealed with Cavit™

(3M, Two Harbors, MN, USA) temp filling material and the temp restoration (Unifast® III, GC Corporation, Tokyo, Japan) was replaced, followed by verification of the occlusion.

Second visit (Day 25): The Pt reported that his condition had improved but he continued to experience discomfort. The redness around his gingiva had resolved. However, sensitivity to percussion and palpation for teeth #3 and #4 remained. Local anesthesia was administrated by infiltration of 1.8 ml of 2% xylocaine with 1:80,000 epi. The temp restoration was removed, RDI was placed, and the tooth was re-accessed. The pulp chamber was irrigated with 5% NaOCl; purulence or secretion of other fluids was not observed. The canal was excessively enlarged and the master apical file was set at size #90. The canal was irrigated with 5% NaOCl and then dried with sterile paper points. Ca(OH)$_2$ was administered into the canal, access was sealed with Cavit™ temp filling material, and the temp restoration was replaced.

Third visit (Day 39): The Pt presented asymptomatic (ASX) with no apical tenderness or percussion sensitivity for teeth #3 and #4. Local anesthesia was performed by injecting 1.8 ml of 2% xylocaine with 1:80,000 epi, and the temp restoration was removed. RDI was placed and the tooth was re-accessed. The canal was irrigated with 5% NaOCl and 15% ethylenediaminetetraacetic acid (Morhonine®, Showa Yakuhin Kako, Tokyo, Japan). The WL and diameter were re-established. The canal was dried and obturated using laterally condensation technique (Figures 17.3 and 17.4). Access was sealed with Cavit™ temp filling material and the temp restoration was replaced. The Pt was

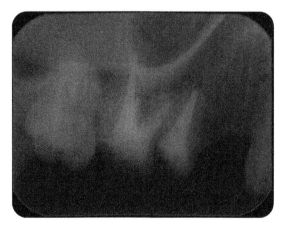

Figure 17.3 Periapical radiograph showing completed obturation of teeth #3 and #4.

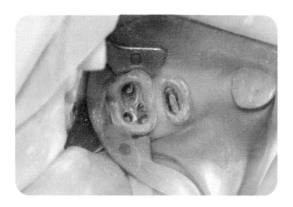

Figure 17.4 Intraoral photograph taken immediately after root canal obturation.

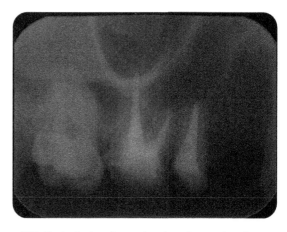

Figure 17.5 Periapical radiograph taken 6 months after root canal treatment.

advised to return to a general dentist for placement of permanent restoration.

Working length, apical size, and obturation technique

Canal	Working Length	Apical size	Obturation Materials and Techniques
Single	13.0 mm	90	AH Plus® sealer, Lateral condensation

Postoperative Evaluation

Fourth visit (3-month follow-up): The Pt was ASX and his soft tissues appeared to be normal. Periodontal probing was within 3 mm with no tenderness to either percussion or palpation.

Fifth visit (6-month follow-up): The Pt remained ASX with normal soft tissues. PA radiography demonstrated osseous healing in progress (Figure 17.5). Periodontal probing was within 3 mm with no tenderness to either percussion or palpation.

Sixth visit (1-year follow-up): The Pt still presented ASX with normal soft tissues. PA radiography demonstrated complete osseous healing (Figure 17.6). Periodontal probing was within 3 mm with no tenderness to either percussion or palpation.

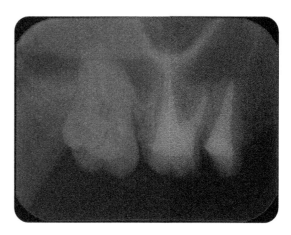

Figure 17.6 Periapical radiograph taken 12 months after root canal treatment.

Addendum

Due to the objective, this chapter does not provide a detailed description of tooth #3. However, tooth #3 also received non-surgical endodontic treatment at this time under the following diagnosis.

Pulpal

Previously initiated therapy, tooth #3

Apical

Symptomatic Apical Periodontitis, tooth #3

Tooth #3 was also asymptomatic after RCT.

Self-Study Questions

A. What is the number of root canals in maxillary/mandibular premolars? List all major morphological anomalies associated with maxillary/mandibular premolars.

B. What are the differences between RCT and initial treatment? What should a practitioner be cautious of before starting re-treatment?

C. Is complete removal of previously filled gutta-percha from the root canal possible?

D. What is the success rate of premolar root canal re-treatment? What is the difference in success rate between root canal re-treatment and initial treatment?

E. What condition should a practitioner distinguish from periapical periodontitis before initiating root canal re-treatment?

Answers to Self-Study Questions

A. Anatomical knowledge, including the number of root canals, is important for all root canal treatment, especially when locating the root canal orifice. Table 17.1 presents Vertucci's classification and number of root canals in maxillary/mandibular premolars (Vertucci 1984). Knowledge of the variety of anomalies associated with these teeth is also necessary. For example, mandibular premolars occasionally exhibit dens evaginatus that causes pulpal infection and periapical periodontitis (Cleghorn, Christie & Dong 2007). While rare, mandibular 1st premolars may also present C-shaped canals (Cleghorn *et al.* 2007).

B. One of the fundamental differences between root canal re-treatment and initial treatment is that re-treated teeth contain previously filled material. The removal of this material comprises the first important step of re-treatment protocols. Various methods to remove material have been advocated such as the use of hand files, nickel-titanium rotary files, and ultrasonic instruments with or without the adjunctive use of a solvent.

Moreover, iatrogenic mishaps such as ledge formation, perforation, and broken instruments may have occurred during previous treatment, making sufficient cleaning and shaping difficult to achieve in re-treatment cases.

C. Although one of the aims of re-treatment is to completely remove the previously filled material, the complete removal of all material, including the sealer, remains a challenge (Duncan & Chong 2008).

D. It should be noted that the success rate of re-treatment is lower than that of initial treatment. The success rate of premolar root canal re-treatment (Table 17.2) has been reported to be between 65% and 71.8% (Ng, Mann & Gulabivala 2008), compared with 80.7% and 86.2% with initial treatment (Ng *et al.* 2007). Moreover, re-treatment cases where the tooth has experienced iatrogenic mishaps (e.g., ledge formation) during previous treatment have a significantly reduced success rate compared with cases without iatrogenic difficulties (Gorni & Gagliani 2004).

E. Premolars, especially maxillary premolars, are susceptible to vertical root fracture. Differential diagnosis is necessary before re-treatment is initiated. Common signs and symptoms of vertical root fracture are localized deep periodontal pocket and a sinus tract that is located coronally, close to the gingival margin (Tamse 2006; Tsesis *et al.* 2010). The most frequent radiographic appearance of a vertical root fracture is the "halo" lesion, which is a

Table 17.1 Classification and number of root canals (%) in maxillary/mandibular premolars (Vertucci 1984).

Tooth	Type I 1 canal (%)	Type II 2-1 canals (%)	Type III 1-2-1 canals (%)	Total with one canal at apex (%)	Type IV 2 canals (%)	Type V 1-2 canals (%)	Type VI 2-1-2 canals (%)	Type VII 1-2-1-2 canals (%)	Total with two canals at apex (%)	Type VIII 3 canals (%)	Total with three canals at apex (%)
Maxillary 1st Premolar	8	18	0	26	62	7	0	0	69	5	5
Maxillary 2nd Premolar	48	22	5	75	11	6	5	2	24	1	1
Mandibular 1st Premolar	70	0	4	74	1.5	24	0	0	25.5	0.5	0.5
Mandibular 2nd Premolar	97.5	0	0	97.5	0	2.5	0	0	2.5	0	0

Table 17-2 Clinical outcomes for initial premolar treatment and re-treatment.

	Success rate (%)	
Tooth	Re-treatment	Initial treatment
Maxillary Premolars	65.0	80.7
Mandibular Premolars	71.8	86.2

combination of periapical and perilateral radiolucency surrounding the root (Tamse 2006; Tsesis *et al.* 2010). If any of the aforementioned features are detected at diagnosis, a practitioner should suspect vertical root fracture.

References

Cleghorn, B. M., Christie, W. H. & Dong, C. C. (2007) The root and root canal morphology of the human mandibular first premolar: A literature review. *Journal of Endodontics* **33**, 509–516.

Duncan, H. F. & Chong, B. S. (2008) Removal of root filling materials. *Endodontic Topics* **19**, 33–57.

Gorni, F. G. & Gagliani, M. M. (2004) The outcome of endodontic re-treatment: A 2-yr follow-up. *Journal of Endodontics* **30**, 1–4.

Ng, Y. L., Mann, V., Rahbaran, S. et al. (2007) Outcome of primary root canal treatment: Systematic review of the literature – Part 1. Effects of study characteristics on probability of success. *International Endodontic Journal* **40**, 921–939.

Ng, Y. L., Mann, V. & Gulabivala, K. (2008) Outcome of secondary root canal treatment: A systematic review of the literature. *International Endodontic Journal* **41**, 1026–1046.

Tamse, A. (2006) Vertical root fractures in endodontically treated teeth: Diagnostic signs and clinical management. *Endodontic Topics* **13**, 84–94.

Tsesis, I., Rosen, E., Tamse, A. et al. (2010) Diagnosis of vertical root fractures in endodontically treated teeth based on clinical and radiographic indices: A systematic review. *Journal of Endodontics* **36**, 1455–1458.

Vertucci, F. J. (1984) Root canal anatomy of the human permanent teeth. *Oral Surgery, Oral Medicine, Oral Pathology* **58**, 589–599.

18

Non-surgical Re-treatment Case III: Mandibular Molar

Bruce Y. Cha

LEARNING OBJECTIVES

■ To be able to formulate a correct endodontic diagnosis and optimal treatment plan from clinical assessment and radiographs.

■ To describe and justify the rationale of various treatment options to manage post-treatment periapical disease based on an integrated analysis of dental anatomy and pathobiology.

■ To be able to obtain informed consent from patients based on ethical communication and evidence-based education.

■ To understand the complexity of using advanced diagnostic imaging modalities and treatment devices to deliver non-surgical re-treatment procedures in mandibular 2nd molars.

■ To understand the importance of safeguarding the health of the patient by determining the status of healing at a follow-up visit.

	Molars			Premolars		Canine	Incisors				Canine	Premolars		Molars		
							Maxillary arch									
Universal tooth designation system	1	2	3	4	5	6	7	8	9	10	11	12	13	14	15	16
International standards organization designation system	18	17	16	15	14	13	12	11	21	22	23	24	25	26	27	28
Palmer method	8⌐	7⌐	6⌐	5⌐	4⌐	3⌐	2⌐	1⌐	⌐1	⌐2	⌐3	⌐4	⌐5	⌐6	⌐7	⌐8
Palmer method	8⌐	7⌐	6⌐	5⌐	4⌐	3⌐	2⌐	1⌐	⌐1	⌐2	⌐3	⌐4	⌐5	⌐6	⌐7	⌐8
International standards organization designation system	48	47	46	45	44	43	42	41	31	32	33	34	35	36	37	38
Universal tooth designation system	32	31	30	29	28	27	26	25	24	23	22	21	20	19	18	17
							Mandibular arch									
		Right										**Left**				

Clinical Cases in Endodontics, First Edition. Edited by Takashi Komabayashi.
© 2018 John Wiley & Sons, Inc. Published 2018 by John Wiley & Sons, Inc.

Chief Complaint

"Swelling on the gum near the last molar on the right side of the lower jaw. It is painful to touch. My face is swollen, too."

Medical History

The patient (Pt) was a 72-year-old Caucasian female. She took Synthroid® 0.025 mg daily for hypothyroidism, Meloxicam 7.5 mg daily for arthritis, and Lexapro® 10 mg once daily for depression. She also used an estrogen patch daily and Restasis® drops for dry eyes. She had been taking Prolix™ injections for postmenopausal osteoporosis for ten years.

She had adverse gastrointestinal reactions to penicillin, clindamycin, and Flagyl®. She was a non-smoker and a retired educator.

The Pt was considered American Society of Anesthesiologists Physical Status Scale (ASA) Class II.

Dental History

The Pt started to experience severe pain on tooth #31 and swelling in the adjacent gum tissue during the previous weekend. She also noticed that her face became swollen. Her general dentist put her on Keflex® 500 mg three times daily which made her pain and swelling more tolerable. When tooth #31 had root canal treatment (RCT) about ten years ago, the Pt was told that the tooth had a hairline crack at the distal marginal ridge. The Pt did not remember any specific information related to RCT done for tooth #30. She indicated her anxiety about dental procedures in general and was concerned about potential osteonecrosis of the jaw related to her current medication if the tooth should be extracted.

Clinical Evaluation: Diagnostic Procedures Examinations

Extra-oral Examination (EOE)

The Pt seemed to be in acute distress. The Pt's face was swollen on the right side. Clinical examination revealed lymphadenopathy on the right submandibular area. The body temperature was 98.4° F. The Pt had trismus related to facial swelling. However, the tempromandibular joint was within normal limits (WNL) without symptoms and signs of popping and clicking.

Intra-oral Examination (IOE)

The gum was swollen at the buccal (B) area of tooth #31 and was sensitive to palpation. Tooth #31 was remarkably sensitive to percussion with class 2

mobility. The margin of crown on tooth #31 was intact. Periodontal probing was not performed due to the pain and swelling in the gum.

Diagnostic Tests

Tooth	#31	#30
Percussion	++	–
Palpation	++	–
Cold	N/A	N/A
Mobility	Yes	No
EPT	N/A	N/A
Swelling	++	+

EPT: Electric pulp test; ++: Percussion/ palpation/swelling significant;
+: Swelling exists; –: No response to percussion/palpation; N/A: Not applicable

Radiographic Findings

In the 2-D periapical radiograph (Figure 18.1), there seemed to be periapical radiolucency (PARL) with loss of lamina dura present at the apex of the mesial (M) root of tooth #31. The PARL at the M root extended to the M area of the distal (D) root apex. There was a full crown with amalgam restoration at the M area. A threaded post in the D root showed a 2 mm gap apically to the root canal filling. The root canal fillings in both roots reached 1 mm point from the radiographic apices. Sclerosis of the bone was observed in the periapical bone or the D root of tooth #31 and in the periapical bone of both roots of tooth #30. The D root canal filling of tooth #30 was underextended by 3 mm. Slight crestal bone loss was noticed at the interproximal bone between teeth #31 and #30. Widened periodontal ligament (PDL) and mild vertical bone loss was present at the distal of tooth #31. The furcation was intact on both teeth #31 and #30.

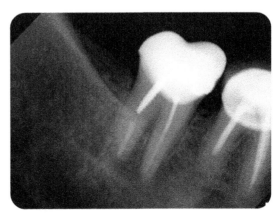

Figure 18.1 Preoperative 2-D radiograph showing hint of periapical radiolucency mesial root of tooth #31.

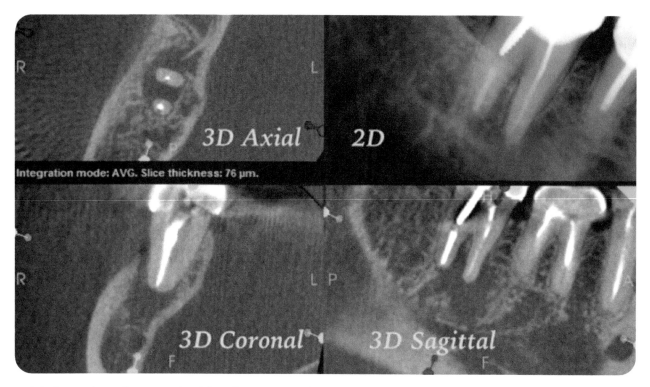

Figure 18.2 Comparison of preoperative 2-D radiograph and 3-D CBCT image showing the enhanced clarity of the periapical in 3-D CBCT imaging.

In the limited-view 3-D cone beam-computed tomography (CBCT) image (Figure 18.2) taken with Kodak 9000 3-D System field of view 50 × 37 mm at voxel size 76 µm (Carestream, Rochester, NY, USA), all axial, sagittal, and coronal slices of each scan were evaluated with the software provided with the CBCT unit. Scans were viewed in a clinical environment on 24-inch monitors (resolution 1920 × 1200 at 60 Hz). Axial, sagittal, and coronal images of each root were examined by aligning the slicing line parallel to the long axes of each canal. In axial view, a definite radiolucency with diffuse border and a diameter of 9 mm circumscribing the M root apex was noticed. The coronal part of the root canal filling in the M root was located slightly off-center towards the B aspect. In sagittal view, the distal border of the radiolucency extended to the D root of tooth #31 and to the inferior border of the lesion encroached to the inferior alveolar nerve canal. The coronal view confirmed the proximity of the lesion to the inferior alveolar nerve which was located 8 mm apical from the apex of the M root. The coronal portion of the root canal filling in the M root was located off-center towards the B aspect as in axial view. In the coronal part, radiolucent canal space suggestive of previously untreated mesiolingual (ML) canal was visible lingual (L) to the root canal filling. In the apical part, the gutta-percha (GP) filling was located in the center of the root in buccolingual (BL) dimension, which suggested merging of MB and ML canals to form one apical foramen. The periapical tissue of both roots of tooth #30 were WNL with normal trabeculation.

Pretreatment Diagnosis
Pulpal
Previously Treated with the exception of ML canal, tooth #31

Apical
Acute Apical Abscess, tooth #31

Treatment Plan
Recommended
Emergency: To obtain drainage
Definitive: Non-surgical (Selective) Root Canal Re-treatment of tooth #31

Alternative
Extraction and dental implant or surgical endodontics

Restorative
Restoration of the endodontic access with amalgam. Replacement of the crown if there is recurrent caries under the crown which compromises the marginal seal.

Prognosis

Favorable	Questionable	Unfavorable
X		

Clinical Procedures: Treatment Record

First visit (Day 1): Anesthesia: 54 mg of 3% mepivacaine was administered for inferior alveolar nerve block (IANB) and 36 mg of 2% lidocaine (lido) with 1:100,000 epinephrine (epi) (0.018 mg) was administered for long buccal nerve block. Dental dam isolation was achieved using Ivory® 12A clamp (Heraeus Kulzer, Hanau, Germany). Indirect visualization was obtained with a dental mirror through the dental operating microscope (DOM; Zeiss OPMI®, Oberkochen, Germany). Endodontic access was made through the metal occlusal surface of the crown. Initial penetration was made with a #2 round bur mounted on high speed handpiece. A Great White™ fissure bur (SS White®, Lakewood, NJ, USA) was used to enlarge the endodontic access, and the M wall of the access was slightly flared occlusally to aid the visualization and the approach of the instruments to the canals. The outline of the endodontic access was shaped as a triangle with a rounded vertex located near the central fossa and the edge of the triangle facing the M marginal ridge of the crown. A surgical length #4 round bur was used in the deeper level excavation of the previous core buildup materials. The visualization of the post and core build up at the D part of the chamber showed no contamination from microleakage. The amalgam restoration at the M area was carefully excavated without water coolant, with air spray to blow off dust which was evacuated with suction for optimal visualization. Slight leakage was seen along the margin of the amalgam restoration. The positions of the chair and the head rest were frequently adjusted to maintain maximum visualization. The B swelling and trismus impaired visualization of the access process, especially for the ML that required the retraction of the DB curtain of soft tissues. A surgical length #2 round bur was used as the excavation process approached the deeper level of the chamber floor in order to minimize unnecessary removal of supportive dentin. The use of the DOM, which provided magnification with illumination powered by Xenon light source, allowed the clinician to discern the subtle difference between the restorative materials and the dentin.

Careful excavation continued with surgical length #2 round bur on the floor of the chamber in search for the orifi of the M canals. In this process, shaving of the dentin layer was followed by air spray for visual inspection. The procedure was executed repeatedly in many small steps in order to avoid accidental perforation of the floor of the chamber and also to preserve dentin. Once the GP in the MB canal was spotted, the search was directed towards the L area to locate the orifice of the ML canal. An endodontic explorer was used to probe the chamber floor in searching for the ML orifice which was discovered slightly L of the GP filling in the MB canal (Figure 18.3). The visual examination revealed dark matter contained in the ML canal. This finding was suggestive of contamination with polymicrobial infection and microleakage. There was a typical anaerobic odor upon discovery of the orifice. The 3-D CBCT image was frequently used as a visual reference in searching for the ML orifice using DOM (Figure 18.4).

The contaminated root canal space of ML was initially accessed with a size #15 K-file in the coronal portion. The tactile sensation indicated that the ML and the GP in the B aspect were contiguous without isthmus in the mid-root level. Using size #20 and size #25 Hedstrom files, the contamination in the coronal portion of the ML canal was cleaned. Then, size #2 and #3 Gates-Glidden burs were used in both MB and ML canals to secure the coronal access. Chloroform was sparingly applied to facilitate the removal of the GP in the MB canal. A crown-down approach was taken to minimize the

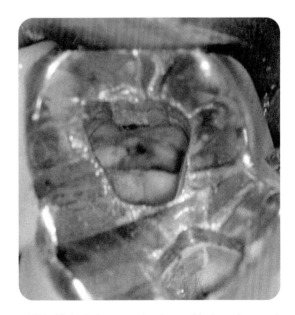

Figure 18.3 Clinical photograph taken with dental operating microscope. View showing contaminated ML canal which was previously untreated. The gutta-percha in MB canal is contiguous with ML canal space. The distal part of the composite core build up with post was intact without leakage. Slight recurrent caries shown at the amalgam restoration at the mesial area.

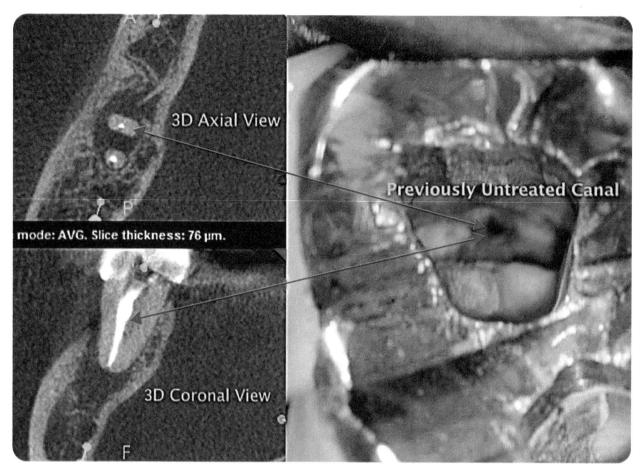

Figure 18.4 The juxtaposition of 3-D CBCT diagnostic imaging and the view through the dental operating microscope (×5.1) correlates the diagnostic imaging with operating field inside the pulp chamber.

iatrogenic irritation to the inflamed periapical tissue. Continued use of Hedstrom files enabled the removal of the GP in MB canal (Figure 18.5). Approaching the apical portion of the canal, working length (WL) was measured with a radiograph taken with a size #25 K-file (Figure 18.6). The determined WL was 18 mm measured on the MB line angle of the endodontic access. Apical patency was checked with a size #10 K-file. There was no drainage coming through the canal.

During the biomechanical instrumentation process, the residues of GP and sealer from the previous treatment were removed with sequential use of K-files and Hedstrom files. Rotary files were also used for the shaping process. 2.5% sodium hypochlorite (NaOCl) and 17% ethylenediaminetetraacetic acid (EDTA) were used as irrigating solutions. An ultrasonic tip (SybronEndo) was used to clean the dentinal walls. The cleanliness and shaped canals were visualized with the DOM after the drying process with size #30, .04 taper paper points. The placement of paper points confirmed the shape of two

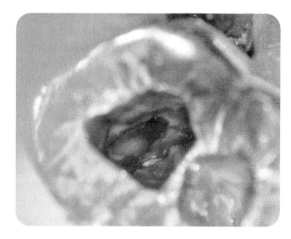

Figure 18.5 Clinical photograph taken with dental operating microscope view after instrumentation and disinfection of ML and MB canals. The gutta-percha in MB canal had been removed.

canals merged to one apical foramen. Calcium hydroxide (Ca(OH)$_2$) was placed in the canals with injection using a 23 gauge needle. A size #30 file was used to spread

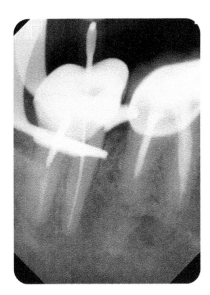

Figure 18.6 Working radiograph measuring the length of the canal.

Ca(OH)$_2$ to the WL. Polytetrafluoroethylene (PTFE) tape was placed over the Ca(OH)$_2$, and Cavit™ (3M, Two Harbors, MN, USA) was used for temporization. After the dental dam was removed, occlusion was checked, including the contact during the lateral excursion.

Performing an incision and drainage (I&D) procedure was discussed with the Pt as drainage was not achieved through the root canal space. The Pt declined to have the I&D at this appointment and was willing to wait and see how the swelling and lymphadenopathy responded in the following 2–3 days. Postoperative (PO) care information was given. The Pt was instructed to continue with the current antibiotic regimen of Keflex. Ibuprofen 600 mg was prescribed on an as needed basis for PO discomfort.

Second visit (Day 16): Pt presented with comfortable condition in tooth #31. With swelling fully reduced, she complained of mild tightness of the muscle on the B area from the previous swelling. There was no pocket probing more than 3 mm. Anesthesia was administered with 54 mg of 3% mepivacaine for IANB and 18 mg of 2% lido with 1:100,000 epi (0.009mg) for long buccal nerve block. Tooth #31 was isolated with a dental dam using Ivory® 12A clamp (Heraeus Kulzer, Wehrheim, Germany). Endodontic access was re-established by removing the Cavit™ and PTFE placed in the pulp chamber. Ca(OH)$_2$ was removed with irrigation of 2.5% NaOCl. The mesial canals were cleaned and shaped with the sequential use of K-, Hedstrom, and rotary files according to the established WL. Then, the canals were dried with size #30, .04 taper sterilized paper points. A size #30 master GP cone was fitted to the WL, and its apical termination was verified with a radiograph. First, the canals were filled

with AH26® Root Canal Sealer (Dentsply Sirona, Konstanz, Germany). Then, the master cone was placed, followed by the alternating steps of spreading the space with D-11 and inserting .04 taper fine accessory points. The GP mass was heated with System B™ (Kerr, Orange, CA, USA) in order to facilitate the lateral condensation process. The root canal obturation process was monitored with a radiograph (Figure 18.7). Excess endodontic sealer was removed by cleaning the chamber with 70% alcohol followed by a washing and drying process. After having discussed how to restore the endodontic access with the referring general dentist on the phone, amalgam was condensed in the endodontic access of the crown. After the dental dam was removed, occlusion was checked, a final radiograph was taken (Figure 18.8), and PO instruction was provided. The Pt was instructed to take over-the-counter ibuprofen 200 mg to 400 mg every 4–6 hours as needed for PO discomfort. The Pt made arrangements for the one-year PO follow-up visit.

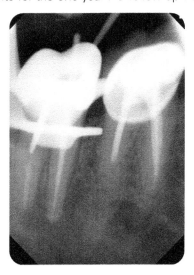

Figure 18.7 Working radiograph monitoring the obturation process.

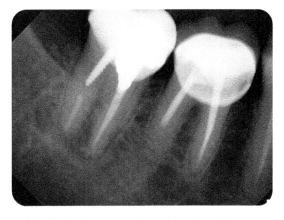

Figure 18.8 Final radiograph taken after obturation of root canal space and restoration of endodontic access.

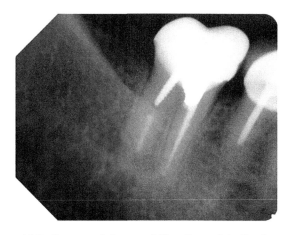

Figure 18.9 One-year follow-up 2-D radiograph indicating complete resolution of the periapical lesion.

Working length, apical size, and obturation technique

Canal	Working Length	Apical Size	Obturation Materials and Techniques
MB	18.0 mm	30	AH26® sealer, Lateral condensation
ML	18.0 mm	30	AH26® sealer, Lateral condensation

D canal was not treated

Post-Treatment Evaluation

Third visit (1-year follow-up): The Pt presented with symptoms of mild discomfort on the right side of the face. She pointed to the region of the right buccinator and masseter muscles. There was no visible facial swelling or submandibular lymphadenopathy. Nevertheless, the muscles were tender on palpation. Tooth #31 was negative for percussion and palpation sensitivity. There was no swelling in the adjacent gingival tissue. The condition of tooth #31 was determined to be stable. The Pt was reassured of no recurrence of periapical infection and informed that the symptoms might indicate possible bruxism or clenching habit. One-year follow-up 2-D periapical radiograph indicated complete resolution of the periapical lesion (Figure 18.9).

Fourth visit (2-year follow-up): The Pt reported no symptoms associated with tooth #31. The crown and the amalgam restoration in the endodontic access were intact. Tooth #31 showed no signs of sensitivity to percussion and palpation. The right buccinator and masseter muscles were not tender on palpation. There was no swelling in the adjacent gingival tissue. Probing depth was less than 3 mm including the furcation area revealed complete healing of the previous radiolucency with uniform PDL and sclerosis of the periapical bone. The follow-up 3-D CBCT image (Figure 18.10) also revealed complete osseous healing of the periapical tissue of tooth #31. The periapical tissue of the D root was also intact in both imaging modalities.

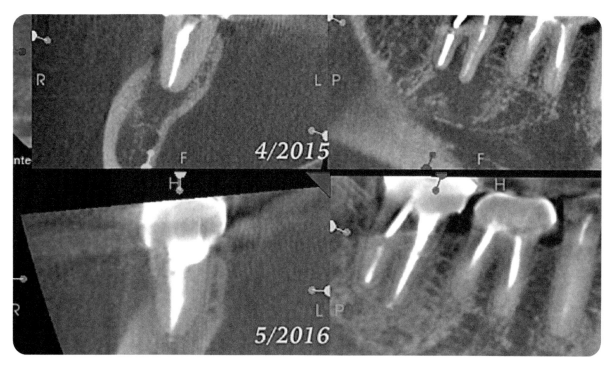

Figure 18.10 Comparison of 3-D CBCT images taken preoperatively (top) and at 1-year follow-up (bottom) showing complete osseous healing of the periapical lesion.

Self-Study Questions

A. What anatomical limitations should a clinician consider when choosing the most optimal treatment option for mandibular 2nd molars with post-treatment periapical disease?

B. What is the rationale for performing non-surgical endodontic re-treatment?

C. How does 3-D CBCT imaging aid in diagnosis and treatment planning for mandibular 2nd molar with post-treatment disease?

D. Why would a clinician choose to perform re-treatment selectively rather than for all the roots of the tooth?

E. How do the procedural steps involved in non-surgical re-treatment differ from initial non-surgical root canal treatment?

Answers to Self-Study Questions

A. Generally, when initial root canal treatment results in post-treatment disease, there are four basic treatment options (Roda & Gettleman 2016):
1. Do nothing
2. Extraction
3. Non-surgical re-treatment
4. Surgical treatment – Periapical surgery, replantation, etc.

There are multitudes of factors that clinicians should consider before choosing the most optimal treatment option. The patient's medical condition, anatomical limitations, the tooth's restorability, and functional value of the tooth are fundamental elements. Favorable outcome depends on the successful elimination of the cause of the post-treatment disease.

Doing nothing does not resolve the post-treatment disease. Clinicians should respect the patient's decision but inform the patient of the risks of non-treatment, including possible progression to more advanced stages of the disease. Clinicians should advise the patient to treat the problem in a way protective of their systemic health. The patient's decision should be documented in the record.

Extraction of a mandibular 2nd molar can cause loss of function. A bridge can be placed if there is a well erupted 3rd molar in the distal area with good plaque control. However, bridge construction is usually problematic due to a short clinical crown. A dental implant can be the most optimal treatment option in restoring the function, provided that the patient is not medically compromised for surgical procedures. Patients who have taken bisphosphonates for osteoporosis need to be evaluated for potential development of osteonecrosis of the jaw after extraction (Advisory Task Force 2007). The location of the inferior alveolar canal can be a limiting factor in proper placement of a dental implant.

Mandibular 2nd molars are the most frequently cracked teeth because of functional and parafunctional stress. Cracked teeth restored via root canal treatment with periodontal probing depth of more than 6 mm is a significant prognostic factor for extraction (Kang,

Kim & Kim 2016). If there is a parafunctional habit, an occlusal guard should be provided to minimize the stress that contributes to cracks.

Non-surgical re-treatment can be an excellent treatment modality when there is a reasonable probability of securing full access to the canals to eliminate the intraradicular microbial pathogens. However, insufficient working space in the posterior mandible can make this treatment option challenging. In the mandibular 2nd molar, accessing the mesial canal is more difficult than accessing the distal canal due to the angle of the canals in relationship with the line of sight of the operating clinician. Clinical conditions, such as acute infection, temporomandibular dysfunction, and trismus, can further impair the clinician's ability to access the canals of the mandibular 2nd molar.

In mandibular 2nd molars, the option of periapical surgery is generally prohibitive due to the thickness of the buccal cortical plate and the location of the inferior alveolar nerve (Burklein, Grund & Schafer 2015). Preoperative CBCT analysis can be helpful to survey the anatomical structure. With the risks imposed by anatomical structure, intentional replantation can be considered if root morphology is in merged shape which makes the replantation process more amenable.

Finally, clinicians should assess their own skill set to meet the level of difficulty before deciding to initiate any treatment modality. "Do no harm" is a critical ethical standard that every clinician subscribes to. If the case exceeds the clinician's level of expertise, referral to a specialist should be an option in order to safeguard or advance the welfare of the patients (American Dental Association 2016).

B. The rationale of root canal treatment remains unequivocally consistent in treatment of primary apical periodontitis or post-treatment periapical disease. Eliminating pathogens and preventing them from re-establishing in the root canal space is the principal goal of root canal treatment.

Intraradicular biofilms are generally observed in the apical segment of approximately 80% of the root canals of teeth with primary or post-treatment apical periodontitis (Siqueira & Rocas 2016). Procedural errors, such as a missed canal, a poorly negotiated canal, ledges, separation of instrument, an obstructed canal, or a poorly obturated canal, can contribute to persistent infection-harboring micro-organisms in the complex canal system. Provided that the canal space can be fully accessed and negotiated, non-surgical re-treatment has a strong advantage in elimination of the intraradicular biofilm over surgical endodontic treatment. From a long-term perspective, the outcome of non-surgical re-treatment is higher than endodontic surgery (Torabinejad *et al.* 2009).

In the case of retreating roots with a missed canal and periapical radiolucency, the procedure should be regarded as initial root canal treatment rather than re-treatment, since the canal was never treated previously. The correct outcome estimate of re-treatment of a missed canal should be 86%, identical to the outcome of initial non-surgical root canal treatment of necrotic pulp with periapical radiolucency (Sjogren, Hagglund & Sundqvist 1990).

Micro-organisms can be also reintroduced to the root canal system through microleakage. The source of the microleakage should be identified and removed. During the course of non-surgical re-treatment, defective restorations and hidden recurrent caries can be identified and removed to prevent microleakage.

C. When the etiology of the diagnosis is identified, the choice of treatment option becomes clear. Clinicians' decisions are bound by the quality of the diagnostic information available to them. 3-D CBCT image is not only superior in detecting periapical lesions, but offers 3-D perspectives of the morphology of the tooth and the adjacent anatomical structure. It is important to notice that treatment plan modification was made in approximately 62% of the cases when additional information was provided by preoperative CBCT imaging (Ee, Fayad & Johnson 2014).

In the case of non-surgical re-treatment, clinicians can locate the canals that were not treated with previous root canal treatment accurately. According to Karabucak *et al.* (2016), the overall incidence of missed canals is 23%. The maxillary molars had the highest incidence (40.1%) of missed canals. MB2 was the most frequently missed canal in maxillary molars. In mandibular 1st molars, 65% of missed canals were second distal canal. 78% of missed canals in mandibular 2nd molars were in the mesial root. The prevalence of apical lesion in teeth with missed canal was 82.8%. A tooth with a missed canal was 4.38 times more likely to be associated with a lesion.

A CBCT image can also provide information on navigating through the canal space, showing findings such as calcification, separated instrument, bifurcation, or dilaceration. Additional information on the location of the inferior alveolar nerve or the relationship with the maxillary sinus floor can be vital in detecting the extent of the periapical pathology and setting the safe boundaries of the endodontic treatment.

D. With the use of 3-D CBCT imaging and dental operating microscope, clinicians are able to accurately identify the root and navigate the root canal space with higher precision. For example, in cases of multirooted teeth such as mandibular 2nd molars, clinicians can isolate and limit the re-treatment(s) on root(s) clearly showing periapical pathosis (Nudera 2015). By carrying out re-treatment procedures targeting those roots with definite problems, clinicians can avoid performing unnecessary and potentially damaging re-treatment procedures in otherwise healthy roots. This selective approach can help resolve the clinical problems with effective precision while minimizing the risks of non-surgical re-treatment procedures such as perforation or fracture.

E. Even though initial non-surgical root canal treatment and non-surgical re-treatment share the identical principle, prevention of re-establishment of pathogens after their elimination from the root canal space, the difference between them lies in the presence of previous treatment.

The patient often asks why the initial root canal treatment did not work and how the non-surgical re-treatment will work. In educating the patient regarding the rationale and strategy of non-surgical re-treatment, clinicians should focus on the facts discovered in the diagnostic process and how to achieve the treatment objectives. Clinicians should refrain from making any judgmental comments about the work that had been rendered previously.

In non-surgical re-treatment, uncertainties of managing the potential presence of undetected perforation, ledges, resorptions, calcified canals, separated instrument, types of existing root filling materials, and/or fracture exist at a higher level.

The difficulties of making access through sophisticated restorations and disassembling of post and core can make the re-treatment process more time consuming and tedious than initial endodontic treatment procedures. These inherent higher risks and difficulties associated with non-surgical re-treatment require an advanced level of clinical expertise and greater understanding on the patient's part.

References

Advisory Task Force on Bisphosphonate-Related Osteonecrosis of the Jaws, American Association of Oral and Maxillofacial Surgeons (2007) Position paper on bisphosphonate-related osteonecrosis of the jaws. *Journal of Oral and Maxillofacial Surgery* **65**, 369–376.

American Dental Association. (2016) *Principles of Ethics and Code of Professional Conduct*. Chicago: American Dental Association.

Burklein, S., Grund, C. & Schafer, E. (2015) Relationship between root apices and the mandibular canal: A cone beam computed tomographic analysis in a German population. *Journal of Endodontics* **41**, 1696–1700.

Ee, J., Fayad, M. I. & Johnson, B. R. (2014) Comparison of endodontic diagnosis and treatment planning decisions using cone-beam volumetric tomography versus periapical radiography. *Journal of Endodontics* **40**, 910–916.

Kang, S. H., Kim, B. S. & Kim, Y. (2016) Cracked teeth: Distribution, characteristics, and survival after root canal treatment. *Journal of Endodontics* **42**, 557–562.

Karabucak, B., Bunes, A., Chehoud, C. *et al.* (2016) Prevalence of apical periodontitis in endodontically treated premolars and molars with untreated canals: A cone-beam computed tomographic study. *Journal of Endodontics* **42**, 538–541.

Nudera, W. J. (2015) Selective root retreatment: A novel approach. *Journal of Endodontics* **41**, 1382–1388.

Roda, R. S. & Gettleman, B. H. (2016) Nonsurgical retreatment. In: *Cohen's Pathways of the Pulp* (eds. K. M. Hargreaves & L. H. Berman), 10th edn, pp. 331. Philadelphia, PA: Elsevier Saunders.

Sjogren, U., Hagglund, B. & Sundqvist, G. (1990) Factors affecting the long-term results of endodontic treatment. *Journal of Endodontics* **16**, 498–504.

Siqueira, J. F. & Rocas, I. N. (2016) Microbiology of endodontic infections. In: *Cohen's Pathways of the Pulp* (eds. K. M. Hargreaves & L. H. Berman), 10th edn, pp. 599–620. Philadelphia, PA: Elsevier Saunders.

Torabinejad, M., Corr, R., Handsides, R. et al. (2009) Outcomes of nonsurgical retreatment and endodontic surgery: A systematic review. *Journal of Endodontics* **35**, 930–937.

19

Periapical Surgery Case I: Maxillary Premolar

Pejman Parsa

LEARNING OBJECTIVES
- To understand the indications and goals for endodontic microsurgery.
- To understand the differences between traditional and contemporary microsurgical endodontics.
- To understand the techniques and materials used in contemporary endodontic microsurgery.
- To understand how microsurgical techniques can enhance the predictability and success of retrograde endodontic therapy, and the potential complications of the treatment.

	Molars			Premolars		Canine	Incisors				Canine	Premolars		Molars		
							Maxillary arch									
Universal tooth designation system	1	2	3	4	5	6	7	8	9	10	11	12	13	14	15	16
International standards organization designation system	18	17	16	15	14	13	12	11	21	22	23	24	25	26	27	28
Palmer method	8⌋	7⌋	6⌋	5⌋	4⌋	3⌋	2⌋	1⌋	⌊1	⌊2	⌊3	⌊4	⌊5	⌊6	⌊7	⌊8

Palmer method	8⌉	7⌉	6⌉	5⌉	4⌉	3⌉	2⌉	1⌉	⌈1	⌈2	⌈3	⌈4	⌈5	⌈6	⌈7	⌈8
International standards organization designation system	48	47	46	45	44	43	42	41	31	32	33	34	35	36	37	38
Universal tooth designation system	32	31	30	29	28	27	26	25	24	23	22	21	20	19	18	17
							Mandibular arch									
	Right										**Left**					

Chief Complaint

"I had a root canal re-done on this tooth and I am still having pain when I chew with it."

Medical History

The patient (Pt) was a 26-year-old Caucasian male. He had no known drug allergies (NKDA). Vital signs were: blood pressure (BP) 122/84 mmHg right arm seated (RAS), respiratory rate (RR) 18 breaths per minute and regular, pulse 72 beats per minute (BPM) and regular.

The Pt was American Society of Anesthesiologists Physical Status Scale (ASA) Class I.

Dental History

The Pt had tooth #12 treated with root canal therapy (RCT) and restorative composite 5–7 years prior. The tooth became symptomatic and it was re-treated. After re-treatment, the Pt experienced postoperative pain for a few weeks and it was decided that apical microsurgery should be performed.

Clinical Evaluation (Diagnostic Procedures)
Examinations
Extra-oral Examination (EOE)

Clinical examination revealed no lymphadenopathy of the submandibular and neck areas. Perioral and intra-oral soft tissue appeared normal. Extra-oral soft tissues appeared satisfactory in color and texture. The temporomandibular joint showed no popping/clicking or deviation on opening and was otherwise asymptomatic (ASX).

Intra-oral Examination (IOE)

The intra-oral soft tissue examination had normal appearance, but the root apex had tenderness upon palpation and percussion tenderness was noted (Figure 19.1).

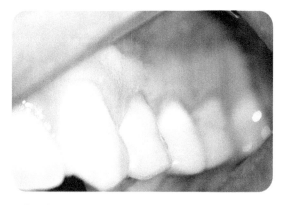

Figure 19.1 Preoperative photograph of tooth #12.

Diagnostic Tests

Tooth	#11	#12	#13
Percussion	–	++	–
Palpation	–	++	–
Endo Ice®	+	–	+
EPT	+	–	+

EPT: Electric pulp test; ++: Severe response; +: Normal response; –: Lack of response

Radiographic Findings

Tooth #12 showed dense root canal obturation with possible extrusion of gutta-percha (GP)/sealer into the periapical (PA) tissues. No final crown was present, but adequate composite restoration and glass ionomer material were placed within access and cavosurface. Tooth #11 was clinically intact without any restorations. Tooth #13 had a mesial-occlusal composite. Tooth #14 had previous RCT with incomplete root filling, but no PA pathosis was noted (Figure 19.2).

Pretreatment Diagnosis:
Pulpal

Previously treated, tooth #12

Apical

Symptomatic Apical Periodontitis, tooth #12

Treatment Plan
Recommended

Emergency: None
Definitive: PA surgery to tooth #12 with Root End Filling.

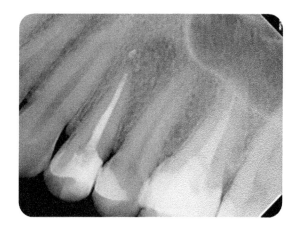

Figure 19.2 Preoperative radiograph of tooth #12.

Alternative

Extraction and dental implant, fixed partial denture, or no treatment

Restorative

Composite or amalgam build up with either onlay or full crown coverage

Prognosis

Favorable	Questionable	Unfavorable
X		

Clinical Procedures: Treatment Record

First visit (Day 1): The medical history was reviewed (RMHX). Vital signs were as follows: BP 122/84 mmHg RAS; pulse 72 BPM and regular; RR 18 breaths per minute. The root tip was assessed based on previous measurements using an electronic apex locator (EAL) (Root ZX® II, J. Morita Kyoto, Japan) from the buccal cusp tip. This helped with creating a precise and conservative osteotomy during surgery. The Tx options were reviewed with the Pt including extraction and no treatment. The Pt elected for apical surgery and informed consent was obtained. The Pt was informed that vertical root fracture might be present. No concerns for anatomic structures were present. The Pt was scheduled for surgery in two months.

Second visit (2 months): RMHX. Vital signs were: BP 118/78 mmHg, pulse 72 BPM and regular. The Pt's mouth was rinsed with 0.12% chlorhexidine for 30 seconds. Anesthesia: two carpules of 2% lidocaine (lido) with 1:50,000 epinephrine (epi) were administered for infiltration, and palatal injections were made to tooth #12 and surrounding tissues. A full thickness mucoperiosteal flap was reflected using an intrasulcular incision from the mesial (M) of tooth #11 to the distal (D) of tooth #13. No apical lesion was present. Based on EAL measurements, a bony crypt was opened 19 mm apically from the alveolar crest using a #4 round bur with sterile saline irrigation. Once the root end was approximated and visualized (Figures 19.3 and 19.4), excess root filling was noted and removed during root resection.

Approximately 3 mm of the root apex was resected using a #171L bur with sterile saline irrigation. The tissue/root end was enucleated from the site. A biopsy was taken and sent to an oral pathologist for review. Hemostasis was achieved using epi pellets within the crypt. Then retropreparations of 3 mm in depth were made into the resected canal using ultrasonic

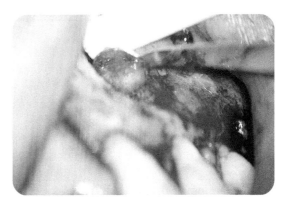

Figure 19.3 Root end inspection and visualization of obturation material with dental operating microscope (DOM)

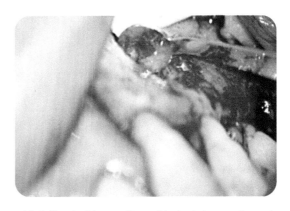

Figure 19.4 Surgical inspection with dental operating microscope (DOM).

instrumentation with copious amounts of water to prevent overheating and potential microfractures of the root surface (KiS 3 tip, Spartan/Obtura™ Figure 19.5).

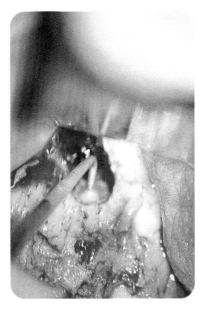

Figure 19.5 Ultrasonic instrumentation (KiS 3 tip, Spartan/Obtura™) in parallel to long axis of root surface and into canal.

The preparation was dried with paper points. White mineral trioxide aggregate (ProRoot® MTA; Dentsply Sirona, Johnson City, TN, USA) Endodontics, Tulsa, OK, USA) cement root-end filling was placed in the root-end preparation and was condensed (Figure 19.6). The surgical site was rinsed with sterile saline. A periapical radiograph was taken to confirm the quality of the root-end filling (Figure 19.7). The wound site was closed with five 5-0 silk sutures (Figure 19.8). Postoperative instructions were given along with the following prescriptions: Peridex™ 0.12% (3M, Two Harbors, MN, USA), rinse twice daily, beginning the second day after surgery for one week. The Pt was also advised to take Motrin® 800 mg four times daily for pain.

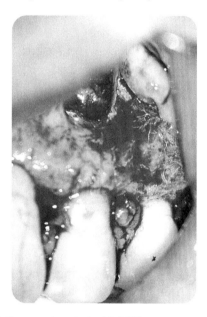

Figure 19.6 Root end sealed with MTA.

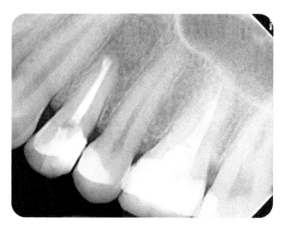

Figure 19.7 Postoperative radiograph of tooth #12 with MTA retrofill.

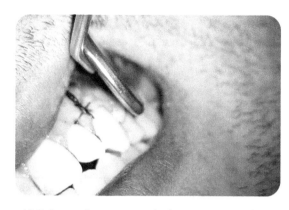

Figure 19.8 Immediate postsurgical appearance, with sutures.

Post-Treatment Evaluation

Third visit (1-day follow-up): A follow-up call was made and mild soreness was reported. The Pt is on Motrin. No other complications.

Fourth visit (1-week follow-up): The report from the histopathologic exam was received. The diagnosis was: Granulation tissue and foreign material. RMHX. BP 125/79 mmHg, pulse 82 BPM and regular. The five sutures were intact and removed without complications. The soft tissue appeared to be healing well. The Pt experienced minimal discomfort.

Fifth visit (14-day follow-up): The Pt reported to be ASX. Soft tissue was healing without complications. There was no percussion tenderness but mild palpation tenderness was noted over root apex (Figure 19.9).

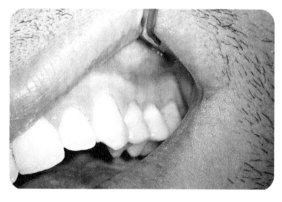

Figure 19.9 Fourteen-day postoperative check.

Self-Study Questions

A. What are some advantages of using cone beam-computed technology (CBCT) during surgery?

B. What are some differences between traditional and modern microsurgery?

C. What is the appropriate management of soft tissue?

D. How much root resection is needed and why?

E. What types of isthmuses are seen during root end surgery?

Answers to Self-Study Questions

A. CBCT offers a great surgical guide for root end procedures. By knowing the correct location of the root end, lesion size, anatomy of tooth, and distance to important anatomical landmarks, the clinician can avoid procedural mishaps and accomplish a complete and predictable surgical seal of the root end. In a study that compared anatomic landmarks using CBCT imaging and periapical radiographs (PRs) before apical surgery, the distance from the lower molars to the mandibular canal could be measured only in 24 of the 64 PR radiographs analyzed (Venskutonis *et al.* 2014). Furthermore, there have been reports that in 70% of cases, CBCT imaging revealed clinically relevant information that was missed by PRs, and bone defects measured on PRs were approximately 10% smaller than on CBCT images (Christiansen *et al.* 2009). Studies also have shown that of 58 detected PA lesions, 15 (25.9%) lesions diagnosed with sagittal CBCT slices were missed with PA radiography (Bornstein *et al.* 2011).

B. Endodontic microsurgery combines magnification and illumination provided by the microscope with the proper use of new microinstruments (Kim & Kratchman 2006). With these new advantages, predictability and precision have increased. The advantages of microsurgery include easier identification of root apices, smaller osteotomies and shallower resection angles that conserve cortical bone and root length. In addition, a resected root surface under high magnification and illumination readily reveals anatomical details such as isthmuses, canal fins, microfractures, and lateral canals. Combined with the microscope, the ultrasonic instrument permits conservative, coaxial root-end preparations and precise root-end fillings that satisfy the requirements for mechanical and biological principles of endodontic surgery (Kim & Kratchman 2006). See Table 19.1 for a brief summary.

C. Previous popular flap designs, such as the semilunar design in the anterior region, are no longer recommended because of scar formation and lack of

Table 19.1 Comparison between traditional and modern techniques.

	Traditional	Modern
Osteotomy size	Approx. 8–10 mm	3–4 mm
Bevel angle degree	65 degrees	0–10 degrees
Resected root end inspection	None	Always
Isthmus identification & treatment	Impossible	Always
Root-end preparation	Seldom inside canal	Always within canal
Root-end preparation instrument	Bur	Ultrasonic tips
Root-end filling material	Amalgam	MTA, Bioceramics
Sutures	4-0 silk	5-0, 6-0 monofilament
Suture removal	7 days postop	2–3 days postop
Healing Success (over 1 yr)	40–90%	85–96.8%

proper access to root end (Kim & Kratchman 2006). Today, esthetics play a crucial role, and the practitioner must minimize any scar formation or recession, when feasible. With modern techniques, flap designs are very similar to those of the traditional techniques: the sulcular full-thickness flap, the muco-gingival flap, and vertical releasing incisions. The once popular semilunar flap design and the Lüebke-Ochsenbein flap design are no longer recommended. In both the sulcular full-thickness flap and the muco-gingival flap designs, the wider base of the flap to improve microcirculatory perfusion was an unnecessary procedure, and it created a lasting scar as a result of cutting the mucosal tissue across the fiber lines. With the current method the base of the flap is as wide as the top, and the vertical incisions follow the vertical blood vessel alignment. This facilitates nearly scar-free healing while still providing more than adequate access to the surgical site. It has been customary to remove 4-0 silk sutures after one week. With the microsurgery technique, mono-filament sutures are removed within 48 to 72 hours for best results. This is enough time for reattachment to take place and the suture removal is easy and painless. After 72 hours, the tissues tend to grow over the sutures, especially with mucosal tissues, and thus removal of sutures may be more uncomfortable (Kim & Kratchman 2006).

D. Studies that evaluate the root apex show that at least 3 mm of the root-end must be removed to reduce 98% of the apical ramifications and 93% of the lateral canals (Kim, Pecora & Rubinstein 2001). As these percentages are very similar at 4 mm from the apex, they recommend root-end amputation of 3 mm, since this leaves 7–9 mm of the root on average, providing sufficient strength and stability. A root-end amputation of less than 3 mm most likely does not remove all of the lateral canals and apical ramifications, therefore posing a risk of reinfection and eventual failure (Kim *et al.* 2001).

E. Five different types of isthmuses have been described. Type I was defined as either two or three canals with no noticeable communication. Type II exhibited two canals that had a definite connection between the two main canals. Type III differed from the latter only in that there were three canals instead of two. Incomplete C-shapes with three canals were also included in this category. When canals extended into the isthmus area, this was named Type IV. Type V was recognized as a true connection or corridor throughout the section (Hsu & Kim 1997).

References

Bornstein, M. M., Lauber, R., Sendi, P. *et al.* (2011) Comparison of periapical radiography and limited cone-beam computed tomography in mandibular molars for analysis of anatomical landmarks before apical surgery. *Journal of Endodontics* **37**, 151–157.

Christiansen, R., Kirkevang, L. L., Gotfredsen, E. *et al.* (2009) Periapical radiography and cone beam computed tomography for assessment of the periapical bone defect 1 week and 12 months after root-end resection. *Dentomaxillofacial Radiology* **38**, 531–536.

Hsu, Y. Y. & Kim, S. (1997) The resected root surface. The issue of canal isthmuses. *Dental Clinics of North America* **41**, 529–540.

Kim, S. & Kratchman, S. (2006) Modern endodontic surgery concepts and practice: A review. *Journal of Endodontics* **32**, 601–623.

Kim, S., Pecora, G. & Rubinstein, R. (2001) Comparison of traditional and microsurgery in endodontics. In: *Color Atlas of Microsurgery in Endodontics* (eds. S. Kim, G. Pecora & R. Rubenstein), pp. 5–11. Philadelphia, PA: W. B. Saunders.

Venskutonis, T., Plotino, G., Juodzbakys, G. *et al.* (2014) The importance of cone-beam computed tomography in the management of endodontic problems: A review of the literature. *Journal of Endodontics* **40**, 1895–1901.

20

Periapical Surgery Case II:
Apical Infection Spreading to Adjacent Teeth

Takashi Komabayashi, Jin Jiang, and Qiang Zhu

LEARNING OBJECTIVES
- To understand the indications for periapical surgery.
- To become familiar with the flap designs for periapical surgery.
- To become familiar with the principles of root-end resection, root-end cavity preparation, and root-end filling.
- To understand the advancements of periapical surgery.
- To understand the success rates in periapical surgery.

	Molars			Premolars		Canine	Incisors				Canine	Premolars		Molars		
							Maxillary arch									
Universal tooth designation system	1	2	3	4	5	6	7	8	9	10	11	12	13	14	15	16
International standards organization designation system	18	17	16	15	14	13	12	11	21	22	23	24	25	26	27	28
Palmer method	8	7	6	5	4	3	2	1	1	2	3	4	5	6	7	8
Palmer method	8	7	6	5	4	3	2	1	1	2	3	4	5	6	7	8
International standards organization designation system	48	47	46	45	44	43	42	41	31	32	33	34	35	36	37	38
Universal tooth designation system	32	31	30	29	28	27	26	25	24	23	22	21	20	19	18	17
							Mandibular arch									
	Right								**Left**							

Clinical Cases in Endodontics, First Edition. Edited by Takashi Komabayashi.
© 2018 John Wiley & Sons, Inc. Published 2018 by John Wiley & Sons, Inc.

Chief Complaint

"I feel pressure and discomfort when I push on my chin."

Medical History

The patient (Pt) was a 25-year-old Caucasian female. Vital signs were as follows: blood pressure (BP) 120/78 mmHg; pulse 68 beats per minute (BPM). No medical illnesses were reported by the Pt, and she was not taking any medication. No known drug allergies (NKDA) were reported. The review of systems was negative.

The Pt was classified as American Society of Anesthesiologists Physical Scale Status (ASA) Class I.

Dental History

Pt had a history of routine dental care. Six months earlier, root canal treatment (RCT) of tooth #24 was completed by Pt's first student provider. A 7x7 mm well-defined circumscribed radiolucency was seen at the apex of tooth #24 (Figure 20.1). Two months later, the Pt presented with severe pain in the lower front teeth. Her second student provider and the clinical preceptor found that percussion and palpation tenderness was more localized to tooth #23. Teeth #23 and #25 were not responsive to Endo Ice® and electric pulp testing (EPT). The periradicular radiolucency (PARL) had enlarged to approximately 17 x 10 mm (Figure 20.2). RCT was started by her second student provider on tooth #23. Upon

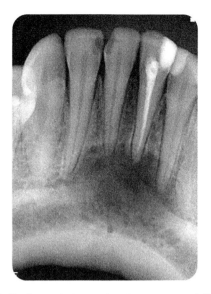

Figure 20.2 Radiograph 4 months after root canal filling of tooth #24. (With permission from Komabayashi, T., Jiang, J., Zhu, Q. (2011) Apical infection spreading to adjacent teeth: a case report. *Oral Surgery, Oral Medicine, Oral Pathology, Oral Radiology, and Endodontology* **111**(6), e15–20.)

follow-up, Pt reported symptoms were relieved after five days. Three days before referral, RCT of teeth #23 and #25 was completed by her second student provider. However, the PARL had continuously progressed (Figure 20.3). Pt complained of feeling discomfort and pressure, especially when she pushed on her chin area. Pt was transferred for further evaluation and treatment (Tx).

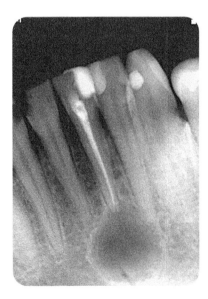

Figure 20.1 Radiograph after root canal filling of tooth #24. (With permission from Komabayashi, T., Jiang, J., Zhu, Q. (2011) Apical infection spreading to adjacent teeth: a case report. *Oral Surgery, Oral Medicine, Oral Pathology, Oral Radiology, and Endodontology* **111**(6), e15–20.)

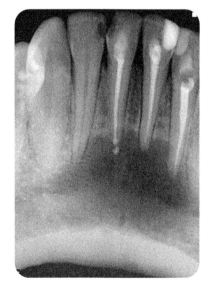

Figure 20.3 Radiograph after root canal filling of teeth #23 and 25. (With permission from Komabayashi, T., Jiang, J., Zhu, Q. (2011) Apical infection spreading to adjacent teeth: a case report. *Oral Surgery, Oral Medicine, Oral Pathology, Oral Radiology, and Endodontology* **111**(6), e15–20.)

Clinical Evaluation (Diagnostic Procedures)
Examinations
Extra-oral Examination (EOE)
Pt felt discomfort from palpation on the chin area. The clinical examination revealed submandibular lymphadenopathy.

Intra-oral Examination (IOE)
Perioral and intra-oral soft tissues appeared normal. Teeth #23, #24, and #25 exhibited mild tenderness to palpation in the labial vestibule. Tooth #24 was restored with composite. The access cavity of teeth #23 and #25 was restored with Fuji IX GP® (GC America Inc., Alsip, IL, USA) glass ionomer cement. Periodontal probing depths around teeth #23, #24, and #25 were 2–3 mm with no mobility.

Diagnostic Tests

Tooth	#22	#23	#24	#25	#26	#27
Percussion	–	Mild pain	Mild pain	Mild pain	–	–
Palpation	–	Mild pain	Mild pain	Mild pain	–	–
Endo Ice®	+	N/A	N/A	N/A	+	+
EPT	+	N/A	N/A	N/A	+	+

EPT: Electric pulp test; +: Normal response to cold or EPT; –: No response to percussion or palpation; N/A: Not applicable

Radiographic Findings
A large ill-defined PARL was seen at the apices of teeth #23, #24, and #25 (Figure 20.3). The lucency measured approximately 20 × 12 mm in diameter and associated with broken lamina dura at the apices of teeth #23, #24, and #25. The root filling of tooth #24 was 2 mm short of apex. Sealer extrusion was seen at the apex of tooth #25.

Pretreatment Diagnosis
Pulpal
Previously Treated, teeth #23, #24, and #25

Apical
Symptomatic Apical Periodontitis, teeth #23, #24, and #25

Treatment Plan
Recommended
Emergency: None
Definitive: Periapical Surgery of teeth #23, #24, and #25

Alternative
Extraction or no treatment

Restorative
Composite replaces the current Fuji IX GP® filling in the access cavity of teeth #23, #24, and #25

Prognosis

Favorable	Questionable	Unfavorable
X		

Clinical Procedures: Treatment Record
First visit (Day 1): During the consultation appointment, the Pt was informed that the continuous enlargement of the PARL with an ill-defined border suggested the periradicular infection had not been controlled despite the RCT on teeth #23, #24, and #25. A Tx plan was presented to Pt including retreatment (re-Tx) of tooth #24, and apicoectomy and root-end filling of teeth #23, #24, and #25. Pt didn't want to have re-Tx performed on tooth #24 because of the RCT experience in the past, with the increasing periradicular lesion. Pt was very concerned with the continuous growth of the periradicular lesion and wanted to proceed with the surgical endodontic therapy as soon as possible. Informed consent was obtained. A prescription was given for Peridex™ (3M, Two Harbors, MN, USA) 16 oz, with instructios to rinse twice daily for two days before surgery.

Second visit (Day 7): Pt had used Peridex™ for two days before surgery. Vital signs were: BP 118/76 mmHg, pulse 72 BPM. Pt was given and took 600 mg ibuprofen for pain premedication. Anesthesia: 36 mg lidocaine (lido) with 0.018 mg (1:100,000) epinephrine (epi) was administered via left inferior alveolar nerve block. 72 mg lido with 0.072 mg (1:50,000) epi was administered as buccal (B) and lingual (L) infiltration adjacent to teeth #22 to #27. A full thickness mucoperiosteal flap was reflected using intrasulcular incision with a #15 scalpel blade from the distal (D) of tooth #22 to the D of tooth #27; two vertical releasing incisions were made at the D of tooth #22 and the D of #27. As the flap was being reflected near the apical area of teeth #23, #24, and #25, significant purulent exudate was evident (Figure 20.4, A). Inflamed periosteum overlaid the purulent filled bone cavity (Figure 20.4, B). Dehiscence of the B cortical bone was seen (Figure 20.4, C). 0.9% sodium chloride (NaCl) was used for irrigation. The bony crypt was

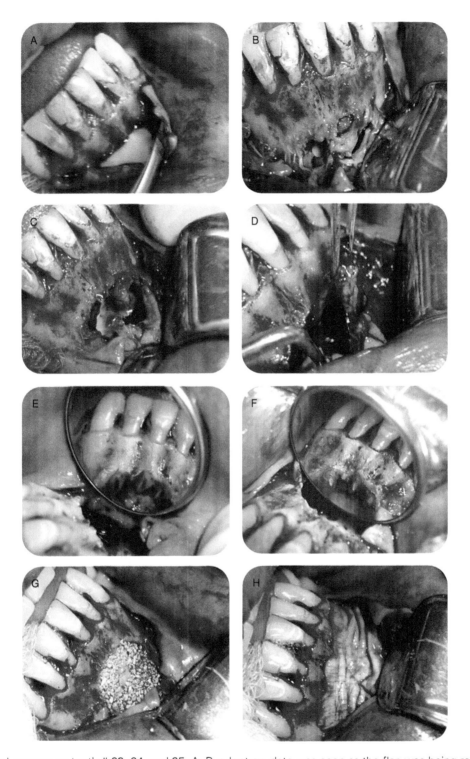

Figure 20.4 Root-end surgery on teeth # 23, 24, and 25. A: Purulent exudate was seen as the flap was being reflected near the apical area of teeth #23, 24, and 25. B: Inflamed periosteum. C: Periradicular lesion. D: Removed tissue attached to the apex of tooth #24 for biopsy. E: Root-end preparation. F: Root-end filling with white MTA. G: Bio-Oss was placed into the bony crypt. H: Bio-Gide membrane was placed. (With permission from Komabayashi, T., Jiang, J., Zhu, Q. (2011) Apical infection spreading to adjacent teeth: a case report. *Oral Surgery, Oral Medicine, Oral Pathology, Oral Radiology, and Endodontology* **111**(6), e15–20.)

modified with a #4 round bur around the dehiscence bone board. Inside the bone crypt a 10x8x4 mm tissue was attached to the apex of tooth #24. The tissue was removed and submitted for biopsy (Figure 20.4, D). Apical 3 mm of the root apices of teeth #23, #24, and #25 were resected using a #171L bur with sterile saline irrigation. The root-end cavity was prepared with ultrasonic instrumentation (Satelec® P5 Ultrasonic Unit, Acteon Group, Mount Laurel, NJ, USA), using a ProUltra® Surgical Endo Tip Size 1 (Dentsply Sirona, Ballaigues, Switzerland). The root-end cavity was dried with paper points (Figure 20.4, E). Mineral trioxide aggregate (ProRoot® MTA; Dentsply Sirona, Johnson City, TN, USA) was mixed with sterile water and placed into root-end cavity and condensed (Figure 20.4, F). 0.75 mg Bio-Oss® (Osteohealth, Shirley, NY, USA) was used to fill the bony defect for effective space maintenance and for promoting revascularization and clot stabilization (Figure 20.4, G). Then Bio-Gide® (Osteohealth, Shirley, NY, USA) resorbable collagen membrane was placed to cover the bony defect (Figure 20.4, H). The membrane served as a matrix for soft tissue support and inhibited soft tissue ingrowth into the underlying bone defect. The flap was repositioned and held in place for about one minute with moistened gauze. Eleven 4-0 vicryl sutures were placed. A postoperative (PO) radiograph was taken (Figure 20.5, A). PO instructions and ice pack were given to Pt. The Pt was instructed to take Motrin® or Advil® 600 mg four times daily for PO pain, and to take Vicodin® when necessary. Prescriptions were given for: Amoxicillin (21 capsules) 500 mg three times a day for infection and Vicodin® (15 tablets: take one tablet every 6 hours when needed for PO pain).

Third visit (Day 14): Pt reported in the first three days she had taken Vicodin® as needed for pain. The 11 sutures were intact. The soft tissue appeared to be healing well except there was a 3 mm area at the end of the vertical incision D to tooth #22 that was slow to heal. The sutures were removed. Pt was instructed to continue Peridex™ rinse.

Pathology report (Day 18): Pathology report revealed a well delineated cyst lined partially by somewhat hyperplastic but non-keratinized stratified squamous epithelium. The wall was somewhat thickened, fibrotic, and contained mild to moderate mixed inflammatory response (Figure 20.6, A and B). The diagnosis was a periapical cyst. However, the clinical surgical finding of a purulent filled bone cavity also revealed a periapical abscess, which could have resulted from the infected cyst originated from tooth #24 or resulted from the root canal infection of tooth #23 or #25.

Fourth visit (Day 20): Pt returned for follow-up. Soft tissue was healing well including the previously

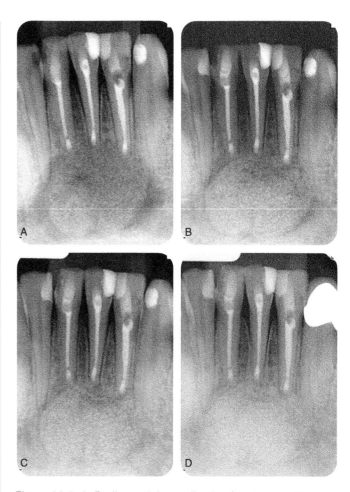

Figure 20.5 A: Radiograph immediately after root-end filling with MTA. B: Six-month follow-up. C: One-year follow-up. D: Two-year follow-up. (With permission from Komabayashi, T., Jiang, J., Zhu, Q. (2011) Apical infection spreading to adjacent teeth: a case report. *Oral Surgery, Oral Medicine, Oral Pathology, Oral Radiology, and Endodontology* **111**(6), e15–20.)

unclosed left vertical release site. The Pt was comfortable, though the labial vestibule was still tender to palpation.

Post-Treatment Evaluation

Fifth visit (6-month follow-up): Pt reported no symptoms. The access cavity of teeth #23 and #25 had been restored with composite. Teeth #23, #24, and #25 were non-tender to percussion and palpation. Probing depths were 3 mm around the teeth. Bio-Oss xenograft material was seen in the radiograph (Figure 20.5, B). Bone fill in the previous radiolucent area was also observed.

Sixth visit (1-year follow-up): The teeth were asymptomatic. Probing depths of 3 mm were present.

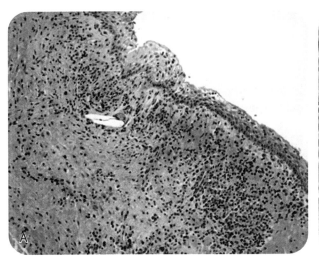 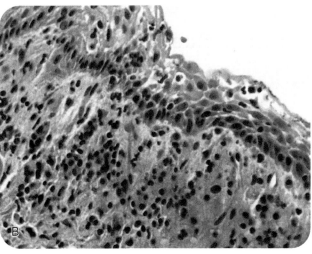

Figure 20.6 Histologic slides of the biopsy tissue revealed a cyst lined by non-keratinized stratified squamous epithelium. The wall contains mild to moderate inflammatory response. A: Original magnification ×10. B: Original magnification ×40. (With permission from Komabayashi, T., Jiang, J., Zhu, Q. (2011) Apical infection spreading to adjacent teeth: a case report. *Oral Surgery, Oral Medicine, Oral Pathology, Oral Radiology, and Endodontology* **111**(6), e15–20.)

Teeth #23, #24, and #25 were non-tender to percussion and palpation. The radiograph showed good periradicular healing (Figure 20.5, C).

Seventh visit (2-year follow-up): Pt reported no symptoms. Teeth #23, #24, and #25 were non-tender to percussion and palpation. Probing depths of 3 mm were present. The radiograph showed the apical lesion had healed (Figure 20.5, D).

Self-Study Questions

A. What are the indications for periapical surgery?

B. What are the flap designs for periapical surgery?

C. What are the principles of root-end resection, root-end cavity preparation, and root-end filling?

D. What advancements have been made in periapical surgery?

E. What are the success rates of periapical surgery?

Answers to Self-Study Questions

A. Indications for endodontic microsurgery are (Kim, Kratchman & Guess 2010; von Arx 2011; Chong & Rhodes 2014):
1. Conventional root canal re-treatment could not be performed or failed (apical lesion develops or does not heal).
2. Persistent symptomatic cases after root canal treatment and/or conventional re-treatment.
3. Conditions require surgical invention such as non-negotiable canals (due to calcification, ledge, transportation, or irretrievable materials in the root canals), perforation repair, material out of apex, and biopsy.

B. The most often used flap is a full mucoperiosteal flap. It is formed by intrasulcular incision along the contours of the teeth with one vertical releasing incision (triangular flap) or two vertical releasing incisions (rectangular flap) extending to the buccal vestibule. The vertical releasing incision should extend at least one tooth anterior and one tooth posterior of the treated tooth. A full mucoperiosteal flap provides excellent visualization and access to the surgical site. The papillary-based flap is designed to preserve the interdental papilla. It prevents papillary recession and is often considered in aesthetically sensitive regions (Velvart, Ebner-Zimmerman & Ebner 2004).

A limited mucoperiosteal submarginal (Ochsenbein-Leubke) flap is formed by a horizontal scalloped incision in attached gingiva with one or two vertical releasing incisions. At least 2 mm of attached gingiva should be retained. This flap is recommended to preserve the gingival margins around crowned teeth. A limited mucoperiosteal submarginal curved (semilunar) flap is a curved incision beginning just beneath the vestibular fold, extending coronally into attached gingiva and curving back into the vestibule. It has limited surgical access and is associated with scar formation; thus, the semilunar flap is not recommended for endodontic microsurgery (Chong & Rhodes 2014).

C. Root-end resection (also called apicoectomy) is the surgical removal of a 3 mm portion of the root end. The purpose is to remove uncleaned apical ramifications and lateral canals. The resected root end is inspected under microscope for possible missed canals, dentin cracks, and isthmuses (Kim & Kratchman 2006; Kim et al. 2010). The root-end cavity is prepared with ultrasonic tips to a depth of 3 mm (Kim & Kratchman 2006; Kim et al. 2010). The purpose is to remove the intracanal filling materials and irritants and create a cavity to receive a root-end filling. Isthmuses need to be cleaned and included in the root-end cavity. A root-end filling places a root-end filling material into the root-end cavity to provide an apical seal. An ideal root-end filling material should adhere to dentinal walls, be dimensionally stable, radiopaque, biocompatible, and without leakage. MTA is the usual choice of root-end filling material due to its biocompatibility and ability to induce cementum formation on its surface (Torabinejad et al. 1997). Intermediate restorative material (IRM) and super ethoxybenzoic acid (super EBA) are also used as root-end filling materials (Chong, Pitt Ford & Hudson 2003; Kim et al. 2016). Recently EndoSequence® BC root repair material and Biodentine® have been introduced as root-end filling materials (Caron et al. 2014; Shinbori et al. 2015).

D. Periapical surgery has been greatly advanced by the introduction of endodontic microscope and microinstruments, especially ultrasonic tips (Kim & Kratchman 2006; Kim et al. 2010; Setzer et al. 2010; Setzer et al. 2012). The endodontic microscope is equipped to examine the operating field with high magnification and focused illumination. The benefits of using this microscope include clear identification of apices, smaller osteotomy, and inspection of the resected root surface for isthmuses, additional canals, and dentinal cracks (Kim & Kratchman 2006; Kim et al. 2010; Setzer et al. 2010; Setzer et al. 2012). The use of ultrasonic tips with the help of the microscope's magnification makes it possible to prepare a 3 mm depth root-end cavity following the long axis of the canal on a shallow beveled root end

(Kim & Kratchman 2006; Kim *et al.* 2010). The advancement of periapical surgery has also been aided by the development of good sealing and biocompatible root-end filling materials such as MTA (Torabinejad *et al.* 1997).

E. Periapical surgery has success rates of over 90% (Rubinstein & Kim 2002; Chong *et al.* 2003; Tsesis *et al.* 2006; Christiansen *et al.* 2009). The Toronto study found the prognosis was better in patients older than 45 years, with teeth having inadequate root-filling length, and with teeth having crypt size smaller than 10 mm in diameter (Barone *et al.* 2010). The meta-analysis studies found the outcome was better when using higher magnification (Setzer *et al.* 2010; Setzer *et al.* 2012) and in teeth without preoperative symp-

toms, teeth with good density root canal filling, and teeth with no or size less than 5 mm apical lesion (von Arx, Penarrocha & Jensen 2010). Teeth with a buccal bone plate more than 3 mm high had a higher success rate than teeth with a buccal bone plate less than 3 mm (Song *et al.* 2013). MTA as a root-end filling material has a higher healing rate than adhesive resin composite (von Arx, Hanni & Jensen 2014) and shows no significant difference compared with super EBA and IRM. Periapical re-surgery also has a very high success rate (93%) (Chong *et al.* 2003; Kim *et al.* 2016). The common causes of failure of apical surgery were no root-end filling and incorrect root-end preparation, that is away from the long axis of the canal and has insufficient depth of less than 3 mm (Song, Shin & Kim 2011).

References

Barone, C., Dao, T. T., Basrani, B. B. *et al.* (2010) Treatment outcome in endodontics: The Toronto study – phases 3, 4, and 5: Apical surgery. *Journal of Endodontics* **36**, 28–35.

Caron, G., Azerad, J., Faure, M. O. *et al.* (2014) Use of a new retrograde filling material (Biodentine) for endodontic surgery: Two case reports. *International Journal of Oral Science* **6**, 250–253.

Chong, B. S. & Rhodes, J. S. (2014) Endodontic surgery. *British Dental Journal* **216**, 281–290.

Chong, B. S., Pitt Ford, T. R. & Hudson, M. B. (2003) A prospective clinical study of Mineral Trioxide Aggregate and IRM when used as root-end filling materials in endodontic surgery. *International Endodontic Journal* **36**, 520–526.

Christiansen, R., Kirkevang, L. L. Horsted-Bindsley, P. *et al.* (2009) Randomized clinical trial of root-end resection followed by root-end filling with mineral trioxide aggregate or smoothing of the orthograde gutta-percha root filling-1-year follow-up. *International Endodontic Journal* **42**, 105–114.

Kim, S. & Kratchman, S. (2006) Modern endodontic surgery concepts and practice: A review. *Journal of Endodontics* **32**, 601–623.

Kim, S., Kratchman, S. & Guess, G. (2010) Contemporary endodontic microsurgery: Procedural advancements and treatment planning considerations. *Endodontics: Colleagues for Excellence.* Chicago: American Association of Endodontists.

Kim, S., Song, M., Shin, S. J. *et al.* (2016) A randomized controlled study of mineral trioxide aggregate and super ethoxybenzoic acid as root-end filling materials in endodontic microsurgery: Long-term outcomes. *Journal of Endodontics* **42**, 997–1002.

Rubinstein, R. A. & Kim, S. (2002) Long-term follow-up of cases considered healed one year after apical microsurgery. *Journal of Endodontics* **28**, 378–383.

Setzer, F. C., Shah, S. B., Kohli, M. R. *et al.* (2010) Outcome of endodontic surgery: A meta-analysis of the literature – Part 1: Comparison of traditional root-end surgery and endodontic microsurgery. *Journal of Endodontics* **36**, 1757–1765.

Setzer, F. C., Kohli, M. R., Shah, S. B. *et al.* (2012) Outcome of endodontic surgery: A meta-analysis of the literature – Part 2: Comparison of endodontic microsurgical techniques with and without the use of higher magnification. *Journal of Endodontics* **38**, 1–10.

Shinbori, N., Grama, A. M., Patel, Y. *et al.* (2015) Clinical outcome of endodontic microsurgery that uses EndoSequence BC root repair material as the root-end filling material. *Journal of Endodontics* **41**, 607–612.

Song, M., Shin, S. J. & Kim, E. (2011) Outcomes of endodontic micro-resurgery: A prospective clinical study. *Journal of Endodontics* **37**, 316–320.

Song, M., Kim, S. G., Shin, S. J. *et al.* (2013) The influence of bone tissue deficiency on the outcome of endodontic microsurgery: A prospective study. *Journal of Endodontics* **39**, 1341–1345.

Torabinejad, M., Pitt Ford, T. R., McKendry, D. J. *et al.* (1997) Histologic assessment of mineral trioxide aggregate as a root-end filling in monkeys. *Journal of Endodontics* **23**, 225–228.

Tsesis, I., Rosen, E., Schwartz-Arad, D. *et al.* (2006) Retrospective evaluation of surgical endodontic treatment: traditional versus modern technique. *Journal of Endodontics* **32**, 412–416.

Velvart, P., Ebner-Zimmerman, U. & Ebner, J. P. (2004) Comparison of long-term papilla healing following sulcular full thickness flap and papilla base flap in endodontic surgery. *International Endodontic Journal* **37**, 687–693.

von Arx, T. (2011) Apical surgery: A review of current techniques and outcome. *Saudi Dental Journal* **23**, 9–15.

von Arx, T., Penarrocha, M. & Jensen, S. (2010) Prognostic factors in apical surgery with root-end filling: A meta-analysis. *Journal of Endodontics* **36**, 957–973.

von Arx, T., Hanni, S. & Jensen, S. S. (2014) 5-year results comparing mineral trioxide aggregate and adhesive resin composite for root-end sealing in apical surgery. *Journal of Endodontics* **40**, 1077–1081.

21

Periapical Surgery Case III: Maxillary Molar

Parisa Zakizadeh

LEARNING OBJECTIVES

- To understand the underlying and contributing etiologic factors resulting in the failure of previous root canal treatments.
- To learn indications and contraindications of apicoectomy on maxillary molars.
- To learn the anatomical landmarks considered during radiographic evaluation of the posterior maxillary region.

- To be familiar with the clinical benefits of using cone beam-computed tomography (CBCT) on maxillary molars when indicated.
- To understand the importance of preventive measures to avoid complications of periradicular surgery/apicoectomy on maxillary molars.
- To learn the correct location of root resection and its bevel during apicoectomy.
- To identify the appropriate changes necessary during resection of root apices to achieve the best results.

	Molars			Premolars		Canine	Incisors				Canine	Premolars		Molars		
							Maxillary arch									
Universal tooth designation system	1	2	3	4	5	6	7	8	9	10	11	12	13	14	15	16
International standards organization designation system	18	17	16	15	14	13	12	11	21	22	23	24	25	26	27	28
Palmer method	8	7	6	5	4	3	2	1	1	2	3	4	5	6	7	8
Palmer method	8	7	6	5	4	3	2	1	1	2	3	4	5	6	7	8
International standards organization designation system	48	47	46	45	44	43	42	41	31	32	33	34	35	36	37	38
Universal tooth designation system	32	31	30	29	28	27	26	25	24	23	22	21	20	19	18	17
							Mandibular arch									
			Right										Left			

Clinical Cases in Endodontics, First Edition. Edited by Takashi Komabayashi.
© 2018 John Wiley & Sons, Inc. Published 2018 by John Wiley & Sons, Inc.

Chief Complaint

"I have a pimple in my gum from which pus comes out from time to time. So far the area has swelled up a few times but after the swelling goes away I have minimal pain."

Medical History

The patient (Pt) was a 53-year-old Caucasian male. His vital signs were as follows: blood pressure (BP) 128/72 mmHg left arm seated (LAS); pulse 71 beats per minute (BPM)/Regular. A complete review of systems was conducted. Pt reported mild seasonal allergies for which usually no medication was required. Pt had no known drug allergies (NKDA).

The Pt was American Society of Anesthesiologists Physical Status Scale (ASA) Class II.

Dental History

The Pt showed an extensive dental restorative history including several composite and amalgam fillings, root canal treatments (RCT), and crown/bridge restorations. His general dentist referred him to see an endodontist for tooth #14 since it had RCT previously and the Pt had occasional discomfort along with swelling in the area. The Pt mentioned that the RCT was done few years ago and he remembered that surgery was done on that area as well but did not remember exactly at what location and whether an endodontist or a general dentist performed the procedure. He experienced mild pain only when swelling appeared. The Pt was interested in saving the tooth.

Clinical Evaluation (Diagnostic Procedures)
Examinations
Extra-oral Examination (EOE)

No edema, lymphadenopathy or asymmetry was present. Temporomandibular joints showed no popping/clicking or deviation on opening and the Pt was asymptomatic (ASX).

Intra-oral Examination (IOE)

The Pt had good oral hygiene with mild staining. In the upper left quadrant (ULQ), distoocclusal (DO) composite on tooth #12, crown restorations on teeth #13 and #14, and occlusal (O) composite on tooth #15 were present. There was a non-patent sinus tract on apical of mesio-buccal (MB) root of tooth #14 with no isolated pocket. The rest of the oral mucosa appeared to be normal with no swelling. Probing depths were 2–3 mm in ULQ except mesiolingual (ML) and distolingual (DL) of teeth #14

and #15 which were 4 mm. No abnormal mobility on teeth noted in ULQ.

Diagnostic Tests

Tooth	#11	#12	#13	#14	#15
Percussion	Normal	Normal	Normal	Mild hyper-sensitivity	Normal
Palpation	Normal	Normal	Normal	Mild hyper-sensitivity	Normal
Cold	Normal	Normal	No response	No response	Normal
Bite	Normal	Normal	Normal	Mild hyper-sensitivity	Normal

Radiographic Interpretation

Tooth #13 had RCT with post/crown restoration. Tooth #14 had previous RCT showing four filled canals and a large/long off-angled post in the palatal canal. Palatal apex looked blunted with wide root filler indicating possible previous apicoectomy or treated wide apex. Apical radiolucency was associated with both MB and distobuccal (DB) roots. The RCT looked acceptable radiographically (Figure 21.1).

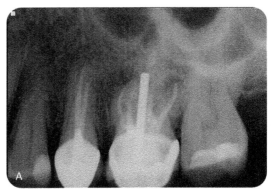

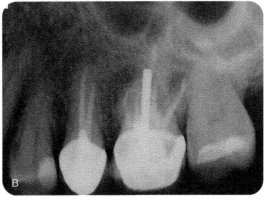

Figure 21.1 Preoperative radiographs of tooth #14 (A and B).

Pretreatment Diagnosis

Pulpal

Previously Treated, tooth #14

Apical

Chronic Apical Abscess, tooth #14

Treatment Plan

Recommended

Emergency: No emergency treatment indicated
Definitive: Periradicular Surgery, Apicoectomy, and
Root-end Fillings

Alternative

Extraction of tooth #14 or no treatment

Restorative

No further restorative treatment required for surgical
root canal treatment option

Prognosis

Favorable	Questionable	Unfavorable
X		

Clinical Procedures: Treatment Record

First visit (Day 1): The Pt presented for consultation
regarding Tx on tooth #14. BP 128/72 mmHg LAS; Pulse
71 BPM/regular. Examinations and diagnostic tests were
performed (Figure 21.1) and a diagnosis was made. The
Pt was Informed of Tx options. The Pt was told that the
RCT on MB and DB roots appeared to be failing. Since
no radiolucency was associated with the palatal root
with presence of a large, long, and off-angled post, the
plan was to explore only the B area surgically. If no
fracture was present, apicoectomy on B roots would be
the Tx of choice. However, follow-up was recommended
on the palatal root. The Pt was scheduled to receive
surgical Tx on B roots at next appointment.

Second visit (5 weeks): The Pt presented for planned
periradicular surgery/apicoectomy on MB and DB roots
of tooth #14. BP 129/80 mmHg LAS; Pulse 60 BPM/
regular; Temperature: 98.9° F; Respiratory rate 24
breaths per minute. The surgical procedure, prognosis,
and postoperative instructions (POI) were reviewed
with the Pt and consent was signed. Anesthesia was
administered with 54 mg 2% lidocaine (lido), 1:100,000
epinephrine (epi), 36 mg lido 2%, 1:50,000 epi, B
infiltration, left posterior superior alveolar nerve (PSA),

and greater palatine blocks. A sulcular incision was
made from mesial (M) of tooth #13 to M of tooth #15. A
vertical releasing incision was made at M of tooth #13
with a #15 blade. A full thickness mucoperiosteal flap
was reflected. Upon reflection of the flap, the
periradicular area of MB and DB roots were exposed,
showing fenestrations over the apical third of both B
roots. The fenestrations were enlarged with a high-
speed round bur under sterile water spray.
Granulomatous tissue was removed using a spoon
currette. The apical region of MB and DB roots were
exposed. No fracture was detected by using methylene
blue and an operatory microscope. Approximately 3 mm
of MB and DB root apices were resected using a #171L
bur. After resection, lack of seal and presence of fin in
both roots were observed. No exposure or perforation
of Schneiderian membrane occurred after enucleation
of all granulomatous tissue in periradicular area. Root-
end preparations made using a diamond ultrasonic tip.
The surgical site was irrigated with sterile saline. Local
hemostasis was achieved by using three epi-pellets in
the crypt and root-end preparations were dried with
paper points. White ProRoot® MTA (Mineral trioxide
aggregate) root repair material (Dentsply Sirona,
Johnson City, TN, USA) was placed at preparation sites
and condensed. Epi-pellets were removed and the crypt
was filled with demineralized cortical bone graft. The
flap was replaced and digital pressure applied for 2–3
minutes. The flap was secured with 4.0 Nylon
interrupted sutures. Good hemostasis was achieved.
A final radiograph was taken (Figure 21.2). POI were
reviewed and an ice pack applied. Favorable prognosis
was expected. An appointment was made for suture
removal. A prescription was given for Peridex™ 0.12%
(3M, Two Harbors MN, USA) with instructions to rinse
twice daily beginning the second day after surgery for

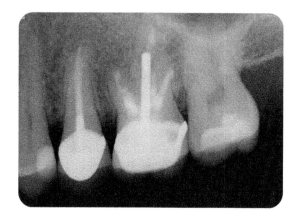

Figure 21.2 Periapical radiograph after completion of apicoectomy on buccal roots of tooth #14.

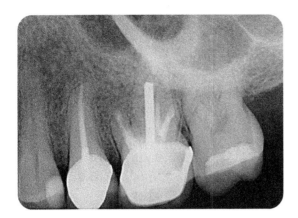

Figure 21.3 Five-week postoperative radiograph of tooth #14.

ten days and to use ibuprofen 600 mg three times daily as needed for pain.

1-day follow-up call: Pt had minimal swelling and discomfort. He was on ibuprofen 600 mg.

Third visit (1-week follow-up): Pt had no complaint of symptoms. Sutures were removed and hydrogen peroxide (H_2O_2) applied to clean the area. The surgical site was healing well without evidence of edema and exudate. Instructions concerning oral hygiene were reinforced.

Post-Treatment Evaluation

Fourth visit (5-week follow-up): Pt was ASX. Periodontal probings were 3–4 mm. No abnormal mobility, sensitivity to percussion or palpation on tooth #14 were present. The radiograph showed healing in progress (Figure 21.3).

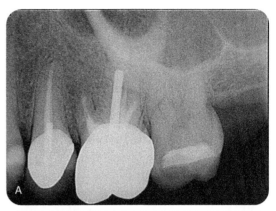

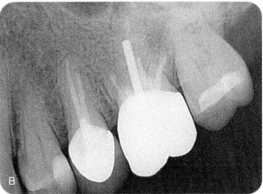

Figure 21.4 Twenty-five-month postoperative radiographs (A and B). Periapical healing is shown on buccal roots of tooth #14.

Fifth visit (25-month follow-up): Pt remained ASX. Upon clinical examination no swelling or sinus tract was detected. The probing depths were 3–4 mm. Follow-up radiographs showed evidence of apical healing associated with both B roots. No apical pathosis was detected on palatal root (Figure 21.4).

Self-Study Questions

A. What are the indications and contraindications to apicoectomy in maxillary molars?

B. What are the anatomical features in the posterior maxillary region that are considered during radiographic evaluation?

C. Is cone beam-computed tomography (CBCT) recommended as an additional tool for planning of periradicular surgery of maxillary molars?

D. What is the best apical bevel of roots undergoing apicoectomy?

E. What is the best approach when the Schneiderian membrane of maxillary sinus is exposed or perforated during periradicular surgery/apicoectomy?

Answers to Self-Study Questions

A. Performing an apicoectomy on maxillary molars is indicated when the following circumstances or conditions exist (Merino 2009; Gutmann & Lovdahl 2011a, 2011b):

- Extremely calcified canals due to aging, trauma and large restorations that prevent negotiating the canal to reach the apical foramen.
- Root canal anatomy (such as extremely curved roots) that is impossible to manage non-surgically.
- An irregular-shaped apical foramen that prevents a complete seal by non-surgical procedures such as apical external root resorptions.
- Failure of non-surgical root canal treatment or persistent apical radiolucencies.
- Reaction to foreign bodies in the periapical tissues such as extrusion of obturation materials beyond the apical foramen.
- Presence of silver cones (Figure 21.5), separated instruments, large/long cast posts or fiber posts (Figure 21.6) which are not retrievable without damaging the root structure.
- Apical transportation, ledges, and zips resulting in root perforations or blockages.
- Post perforations located at the apical third that cannot be treated by non-surgical techniques.
- Necrotic root fragments in horizontal or oblique root fractures that are preventing the coronal fragment from healing.
- Lesions caused by lateral canals at apical third.
- Iatrogenic obstructions.

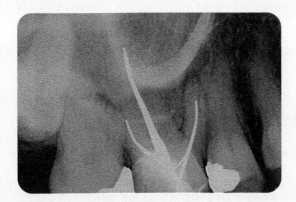

Figure 21.5 Presence of silver cones on tooth #3 with periapical radiolucency associated with MB root.

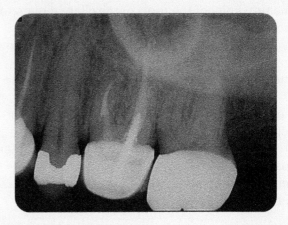

Figure 21.6 Radiograph showing a fiber post placed in MB root with the presence of apical radiolucency on tooth #14. Apicoectomy is preferred on this case over non-surgical re-treatment.

The suggested contraindications to periradicular surgery/apicoectomy on maxillary molars include (Merino 2009; Johnson, Fayad & Witherspoon 2011; Little *et al.* 2013):

- Medical conditions not allowing surgical intervention such as uncontrolled diabetes and hypertension, alcoholism, IV Bisphosphonates, recent radiation, active infectious oral disease, cancer, or blood disorders.
- Insufficient alveolar bone to support the remaining root structure or poor crown-to-root ratio jeopardizing the longevity of the tooth in the long term.
- Significant tooth mobility.
- Non-restorable remaining tooth structure after surgery.
- Defective coronal restoration or coronal leakage as a factor for failure of an endodonic treatment.
- Lack of tooth's importance in prosthetic plan.
- Poor obturation and good prognosis for successful retreatment.
- Surgery causing endo–perio defect with difficult closure.
- Difficult access of the periapical area during surgery.
- Postoperative care compromised or not maintainable.

B. The anatomical features in the posterior maxillary region that are considered during radiographic evaluation are as follows (Johnson *et al.* 2011):

- The proximity of the roots of maxillary molars to the maxillary sinus.
- Zygomatic process and its radiographic superimposition on surgical area.
- The height and architecture of the alveolar bone.
- The convergence or divergence of the roots of teeth to be treated and the proximity of roots of adjacent teeth.
- Presence of lamina dura and periodontal ligament space.
- Length of roots to be treated.
- Tuberosity.

C. CBCT may play an important role in planning for surgical endodontic re-treatment on the palatal roots of the maxillary 1st molar (Rigolone *et al.* 2003). CBCT allows the clinician to calculate the distance between the cortical plate and the palatal root apex, and to discern the presence or absence of the maxillary sinus between the roots in maxillary molars (Patel *et al.* 2016; Figure 21.7). Root morphology, bony topography, existing buccal alveolar bone perforations or fenestrations, and the inclination of roots of teeth planned for surgical intervention can be analyzed and assessed precisely (Nakata *et al.*

2006; Lofthag-Hansen *et al.* 2007; Low *et al.* 2008). CBCT may also aid in the localization of overextended root canal obturation materials, and the localization of perforations and root resorptions. It has been shown that 34% of periapical lesions detected by CBCT were not detected with periapical radiographs. The likelihood of detecting periapical lesions with periapical radiographs was reduced when the root apices were in close proximity to the floor of the maxillary sinus and when there was less than 1 mm of bone between the periapical lesion and the sinus floor. Therefore, CBCT is more sensitive for detecting periapical lesions associated with maxillary molar teeth (Low *et al.* 2008). In general, the information obtained from a CBCT scan in complex anatomic cases may influence the treatment plan and the treatment outcome (Ee, Fayad & Johnson 2014). Use of CBCT may also prevent procedural errors such as perforations to the maxillary sinus, thus improving the management of apicoectomy of roots of maxillary molars. However, CBCT should only be considered when conventional radiographic techniques do not provide adequate information for the diagnosis and management of endodontic problems (Patel *et al.* 2015).

D. Once the apex is exposed, the apical bevel is prepared so that the canal is visible and centered

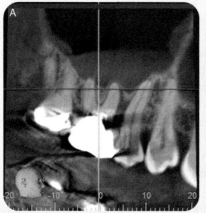 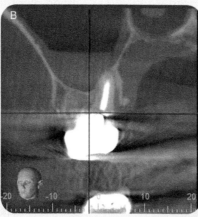 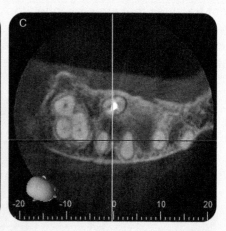

Figure 21.7 CBCT images of tooth #3 with root canal treated palatal root and non-negotiable buccal roots. A: The sagittal image shows the overall extension of maxillary sinus in relation to maxillary 2nd premolar, 1st and 2nd molars. This slice also shows two calcified buccal roots of tooth #3. The coronal slice (B) aids in examining the presence or absence of the maxillary sinus between roots before surgical endodontic re-treatment on tooth #3. In this slice, the interradicular extension of the maxillary sinus in between the buccal and palatal roots is evident. The red line on sagittal (A) image shows where the axial plain shown in (C) was obtained. The axial view also shows the proximity of buccal roots to the maxillary sinus (C).

in the beveled surface. Since 98% of apical canal anomalies and 93% of lateral canals exist in the apical 3 mm, it is important to resect at least 3 mm of the root end (Gutmann & Pitt Ford 1993; Stropko, Doyon & Gutmann 2005). However, if a dye discloses the presence of an accessory canal, a greater length of root must be removed (Roy & Chandler 2007). An ideal bevel would be close to perpendicular to the long axis of the root, in order to decrease dentin tubules peripheral microfiltration (Gilheany, Figdor & Tyas 1994); often 30° or 45° bevels are needed for better access and visualization without compromising tooth structure. If the bevel is too great, there is a spatial disorientation that is difficult to overcome and the root-end preparation and retrofill may fall short of ideal. The smallest bevel possible is favorable, but for posterior teeth, because of anatomy, changes in bevel are inevitable. Once the root has been resected, it should be carefully examined for cracks or fractures as well as for the presence of isthmuses, fins, and anastomoses. These anatomic variations will then dictate the extension of the resection or beveling of the root end (Gutmann & Pitt Ford 1993; Stropko *et al.* 2005; Gutmann & Lovdahl 2011a).

E. In an event of perforation of the Schneiderian membrane, a resorbable membrane can be placed against the membrane and over the perforated area. If the perforation is small, which is usually the case during apicoectomy, repair may not be needed as long as the Schneiderian membrane "folds over itself" (Fugazzotto & Vlassis 2003).

References

Ee, J., Fayad, M. I. & Johnson, B. R. (2014) Comparison of endodontic diagnosis and treatment planning decisions using cone-beam volumetric tomography versus periapical radiography. *Journal of Endodontics* **40**, 910–916.

Fugazzotto, P. A. & Vlassis, J. (2003) A simplified classification and repair system for sinus membrane perforations. *Journal of Periodontology* **74**, 1534–1541.

Gilheany, P. A., Figdor, D. & Tyas, M. J. (1994) Apical dentin permeability and microleakage associated with root-end resection and retrograde filling. *Journal of Endodontics* **20**, 22–26.

Gutmann, J. L. & Pitt Ford, T. R. (1993) Management of the resected root end: A clinical review. *International Endodontic Journal* **26**, 273–283.

Gutmann, J. L. & Lovdahl, P. E. (2011a) Problem-solving challenges in periapical surgery. In: *Problem Solving in Endodontics: Prevention, Identification, and Management* (eds. J. L. Gutmann & P. E. Lovdahl), 5th edn, pp. 325–355. St. Louis, MO: Elsevier.

Gutmann, J. L. & Lovdahl, P. E. (2011b) Problem-solving challenges that require periradicular surgical intervention. In: *Problem Solving in Endodontics: Prevention, Identification, and Management* (eds. J. L. Gutmann & P. E. Lovdahl), 5th edn, pp. 384–417. St. Louis, MO: Elsevier.

Johnson, B. R., Fayad, M. I. & Witherspoon, D. E. (2011) Periradicular surgery. In: *Pathways of the Pulp* (eds. K. M. Hargreaves & S. Cohen), 10th edn, pp. 720–776. St. Louis, MO: Mosby.

Little, J. W., Falace, D. A., Miller, C. S. et al. (2013) *Dental Management of the Medically Compromised Patient*, 8th edn. St Louis, MO: Elsevier.

Lofthag-Hansen, S., Huumonen, S., Grondahl, K. et al. (2007) Limited cone-beam CT and intraoral radiology for the diagnosis of periapical pathology. *Oral Surgery, Oral Medicine, Oral Pathology, Oral Radiology, and Endodontics* **103**, 114–119.

Low, K. M., Dula, K., Burgin, W. et al. (2008) Comparison of periapical radiography and limited cone-beam tomography in posterior maxillary teeth referred for apical surgery. *Journal of Endodontics* **34**, 557–562.

Merino, E. M. (2009) Presurgical considerations. In: *Endodontic Microsurgery* (ed. E. M. Merino), pp. 33–48. London: Quintessence.

Nakata, K., Naitoh, M., Izumi, M. et al. (2006) Effectiveness of dental computed tomography in diagnostic imaging of periradicular lesion of each root of a multirooted tooth: A case report. *Journal of Endodontics* **32**, 583–587.

Patel, S., Durack, C., Anella, F. et al. (2015) Cone beam computed tomography in endodontics – A review. *International Endodontic Journal* **48**, 3–15.

Patel, S., Harvey, S., Shemesh, H. et al. (2016) Non-surgical and surgical re-treatment. In: *Cone Beam Computed Tomography in Endodontics* (eds. S. Patel, S. Harvey, H. Shemesh et al.), pp. 89–99. London: Quintessence.

Rigolone, M., Pasqualini, D., Bianchi, L. et al. (2003) Vestibular surgical access to the palatine root of the superior first molar: "low-dose cone-beam" CT analysis of the pathway and its anatomic variations. *Journal of Endodontics* **29**, 773–775.

Roy, R. & Chandler, N. P. (2007) Contemporary perspectives on root-end management during periapical surgery. *Endo: Endodontic Practice Today* **1**, 91–99.

Stropko, J. J., Doyon, G. E. & Gutmann, J. L. (2005) Root end management: Resection, cavity preparation, and material placement. *Endodontic Topics* **11**, 131–151.

22

Perio–Endo Interrelationships

Abdullah Alqaied and Maobin Yang

LEARNING OBJECTIVES
- To describe major pathways of communication between the pulp and periodontal tissue, and to identify possible etiologies for perio–endo lesions.

- To understand and apply the differential diagnosis of a primary periodontal lesion and a primary endodontic lesion.
- To be able to make an appropriate treatment plan, including alternative therapies.

Clinical Cases in Endodontics, First Edition. Edited by Takashi Komabayashi.
© 2018 John Wiley & Sons, Inc. Published 2018 by John Wiley & Sons, Inc.

Chief Complaint

"I have pain when I bite hard on my tooth."

Medical History

The patient (Pt) was a 38-year-old male. Vital signs were as follows: blood pressure (BP) 109/70 mmHg, pulse 77 beats per minute (BPM), respiratory rate (RR) 18 breaths per minute. The Pt was not treated for any medical condition. A complete review of systems was unremarkable. The Pt was not taking any medications and had no known drug allergies (NKDA). There were no contraindications to dental treatment (Tx).

The Pt was American Society of Anesthesiologists Physical Status Scale (ASA) Class I.

Dental History

The Pt was referred for evaluation and treatment of tooth #30. Pt reported dull pain when biting on tooth #30. The symptoms had started about two months previously but the symptoms were never severe enough to seek immediate dental care. Tooth #30 had an occlusal (O) composite restoration; the Pt did not recall when it was placed. The Pt was missing all the 3rd molars. Pt did not keep regular dental visits with the general dentist (GD) and had poor oral hygiene.

Clinical Evaluation (Diagnostic Procedures)
Examinations

The Pt was well developed, alert and cooperative.

Extra-oral examination (EOE)

Examination revealed no swelling, extra-oral fistula or lymphadenopathy of the submandibular and neck areas.

Intra-oral examination (IOE)

Soft tissue appeared healthy with no signs of intra-oral swelling or sinus tract. No swelling or fluctuance was noted. Pt had minor gingivitis and moderate subgingival calculus. Tooth #30 had O composite restoration, and class I furcation involvement. Pt had several restored teeth without visible caries, recurrent caries or cracks.

Diagnostic Tests

Tooth	#28	#29	#30	#31
Percussion	–	–	+	–
Palpation	–	–	+	–
Endo Ice®	+	+	–	+
Mobility	WNL	WNL	WNL	WNL

Tooth	#28	#29	#30	#31
EPT (Value)	+ (32)	+ (36)	–	+ (35)
PPD (BOP)	<4 mm (+)	<4 mm (+)	<4 mm (+)	<4 mm (+)

EPT: Electric pulp testing; PPD: Peridontal pocket depth; BOP: Bleeding on probing; WNL: Within normal limits +: Response; -: No response.

Radiographic Findings

A periapical radiograph (PA) showed teeth #29–31. Tooth #30 had a furcal radiolucent lesion, widened periodontal ligament (PDL) space around the mesial (M) root, and an internal resorptive defect in the distal (D) aspect of the pulp chamber. Normal PA structure was seen around tooth #29, the D root of tooth #30, and the M and D roots of tooth #31 (Figure 22.1). A bitewing radiograph revealed tooth #30 with deep O restoration. The internal resorptive defect was located about the orifice level of the D canal. Teeth #2, #3, and #31 were restored with no signs of recurrent caries. The remaining teeth were non-carious and non-restored. The bitewing radiograph showed moderate subgingival calculus and minor loss of bone height (Figure 22.2).

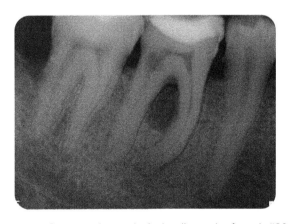

Figure 22.1 Preoperative periapical radiograph of tooth #30.

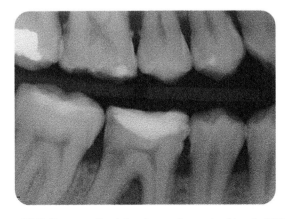

Figure 22.2 Preoperative bitewing radiograph of tooth #30.

Pretreatment Diagnosis
Pulpal
Pulp Necrosis, tooth #30

Apical
Symptomatic Apical Periodontitis, tooth #30
Endo–perio lesion (Primary Endodontic Lesion)

Treatment Plan
Recommended:
Emergency: Pulp debridement, tooth #30
Definitive: Non-surgical Root Canal Treatment
              (NSRCT), tooth #30

Alternative
Extraction and replacement with implant or fixed partial denture or no treatment

Restorative
Post, core and crown

Prognosis

Favorable	Questionable	Unfavorable
	X	

Clinical Procedures: Treatment Record

First visit (Day 1): Upon completion of reviewed medical history (RMHX), EOE, and IOE, treatment options were reviewed with the Pt, who decided to retain the tooth by having a root canal treatment (RCT). Pt was advised that the internal resorptive defect needed to be evaluated during the treatment procedure to evaluate if the tooth was restorable. Pt was aware of the Tx risks and benefits. Informed consent was obtained. Anesthesia was administered with 36 mg of lidocaine with 0.018 mg of epinephrine administered via inferior alveolar nerve block (IANB). Rubber dam (RD) isolation was used and disinfection accomplished. Access cavity and chamber unroofing were completed using a sterile bur. An internal resorptive defect was found in the D lingual (L) aspect of the pulp chamber (Figure 22.3). No bleeding was detected from the resorptive defect. Initial canal instrumentation and negotiation were completed using sizes #8, #10, and #15 K-file. Canal instrumentation was continued under copious irrigation with 0.5% sodium hypochlorite (NaOCl). Working length (WL) measurements were determined using an electronic apex locator and a WL radiograph (Figure 22.4). Coronal flaring was completed

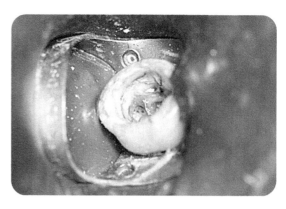

Figure 22.3 Internal resorptive defect was found in the DL aspect of the pulp chamber of tooth #30.

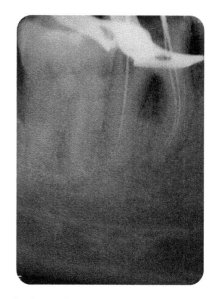

Figure 22.4 Radiograph to measure the working length of tooth #30.

with SX, S1, and S2 ProTaper® Universal files (Dentsply Sirona, Ballaigues, Switzerland) under copious irrigation. Canal instrumentation was completed to size #30, .06 taper master apical file (MAF) for the MB and ML canals and to size #40, .06 taper (MAF) for D canal using EndoSequence® file (Brasseler USA, Savannah, GA, USA). Canals were dried with paper points (PPs). Canals and pulp chamber were soaked with 17% Ethylenediaminetetraacetic acid (EDTA) for 1 minute, dried with PPs, and soaked with 2% iodine–potassium iodide (IKI) for 10 minutes. After the 10 minutes, canals were dried again with PPs, and a slurry of calcium hydroxide ($Ca(OH)_2$) was introduced into the canals using a Lentulo® Spiral Filler (Dentsply Sirona, Ballaigues, Switzerland) and packed with a PP. A slurry of $Ca(OH)_2$ was packed into the resorptive defect as well. The tooth was temporized with Cavit™ (3M, Two Harbors, MN, USA) and Fuji IX GP® (GC America Inc., Alsip, IL, USA).

Occlusion was adjusted. Postoperative instructions (POI) were given to the Pt, who was instructed to take 600mg ibuprofen every 6 to 8 hours (q6-8hrs) as needed (PRN) for pain. Pt was asked to call if symptoms appeared. Pt was instructed to schedule a second appointment to complete the treatment after 7-10 days.

Second visit (5-week follow-up): Pt visited for completion of NSRCT tooth #30: Pt presented asymptomatic. Vital signs were as follows: BP 120/71 mmHg, pulse 81 BPM, and RR 15 breaths per minute. Anesthesia: 36 mg of lidocaine with 0.018 mg of epinephrine was administered via IANB. RD isolation, followed by disinfection. Access was re-established and Ca(OH)$_2$ was removed by copious irrigation with 0.5% NaOCl and minimal instrumentation. Hard structure was evident in the resorptive defect with no signs of bleeding or external communication. Gutta-percha (GP) cone fit was verified with a radiograph (Figure 22.5). Canals were soaked with 17% EDTA for 1 minute followed by 2% potassium iodide for 10 minutes. Canals were dried with PPs. Canals were obturated with GP and AH26® Root Canal Sealer (Dentsply Sirona, Konstanz, Germany) by warm vertical condensation. Alcohol was used to remove excess sealer. The D canal was covered with a thin layer of Cavit™. The resorptive defect and adjacent dentin were etched with 37% phosphoric acid for 1 minute and then rinsed with sterile water. The pulp chamber was dried. A bonding agent was applied and light-cured for 20 seconds. A-3 composite restoration was placed over the resorptive defect and light-cured for 40 seconds (Figure 22.6). The tooth was temporized with Cavit™ and Fuji IX GP® and

occlusion was checked. Postoperative radiographs were taken (Figures 22.7 and 22.8). POI were given. A letter was generated instructing the general dentist (GD) to use one of the M canals if a post and core was needed. The letter was given to the Pt and the importance of permanent coronal restoration and follow-up appointment were emphasized.

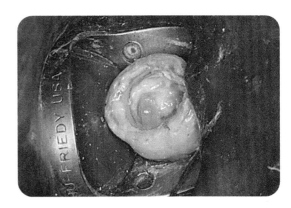
Figure 22.6 Composite restoration was placed over the resorptive defect of tooth #30.

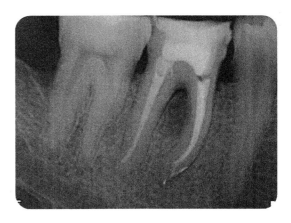
Figure 22.7 Postoperative radiograph of tooth #30.

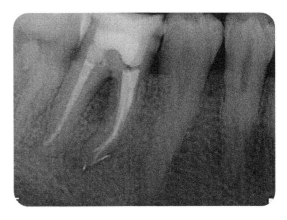
Figure 22.8 Postoperative radiograph of tooth #30 from a different angle.

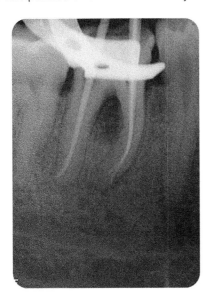
Figure 22.5 Radiograph with the master cones fit of tooth #30.

Working length, apical size, and obturation technique

Canal	Working Length	Apical Size, Taper	Obturation Materials and Techniques
MB	20.0 mm	30, .06	AH26® sealer, Warm vertical condensation
ML	20.5 mm	30, .06	AH26® sealer, Warm vertical condensation
D	19.0 mm	40, .06	AH26® sealer, Warm vertical condensation

Post-Treatment Evaluation

Third visit (1-year follow-up): RMHX. Pt was asymptomatic. Tooth #30 was not sensitive to percussion, and palpation and gingiva appeared normal. PPD was <4mm, there was no BOP, and mobility was WNL. A PA radiograph showed almost complete healing of the furcal lesion. PA radiographs revealed normal PDL space around the M root (Figure 22.9). Pt stated that the GD restored the tooth within two months of the completion of NSRCT. He did not report back for placement of permanent crown. Tooth #30 had post, core and temporary crown. Pt was instructed to get the tooth permanently restored to avoid complications. Prognosis was favorable. Pt was advised to schedule another follow-up appointment to monitor healing.

Fourth visit (20-month follow-up): RMHX. Pt was asymptomatic. Tooth #30 was not sensitive to percussion and palpation. Gingiva appeared normal. PPD was <4mm, no BOP and mobility was WNL. A PA

radiograph showed almost complete healing of the furcal lesion (possible scar tissue) and normal PA tissue. Tooth #30 had post, core and a well-fitting crown (Figure 22.10).

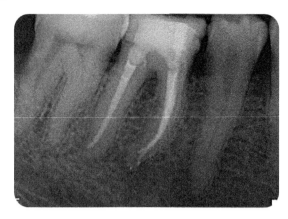

Figure 22.9 One-year follow-up radiograph of tooth #30.

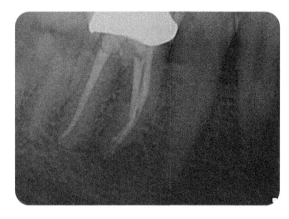

Figure 22.10 Twenty-month follow-up radiograph of tooth #30.

Self-Study Questions

A. List the major pathways of communication between the pulp and periodontium tissue.

B. Describe how pulpal pathosis works as a cause of periodontal disease in the case of a primary endodontic lesion with secondary periodontal involvement.

C. What is the true combined endo–perio lesion?

D. Explain the differential diagnosis used in determining whether a lesion is endo or perio in origin, including both clinical and radiographic factors.

E. In addition to conventional endodontic and periodontal treatment, what are the alternative approaches that can be used to treat the lesions with combined endodontic and periodontal causes?

Answers to Self-Study Questions

A. The possible pathways of communication between pulp and periodontium tissues include: apical foramina (main direct communication); lateral and accessory canals (most often located at the apical third of the root); dentinal tubules; furcation canals; developmental abnormality (e.g., palatogingival grooves on incisors); and pathological or iatrogenic communications, including root resorption, vertical root fracture, and perforation (Seltzer, Bender & Ziontz 1963; Withers et al. 1981).

B. Canal debris, bacteria and bacterial byproducts can spread from the canal system to periodontium through the pathways described in answer A. In addition, during root canal therapy, the process of instrumentation, irrigation and placement of medicament may cause the extrusion of bacteria/ bacterial byproduct, irrigant or medicament beyond the apical foramen. The spread of these irritants may potentially aggravate the periodontal tissue. The above factors can cause inflammation or an infection process in the periodontium. If the pathogens overcome the host defense mechanism, it will lead to the destruction or loss of periodontal tissue (Blomlof, Lengheden & Linskog 1992; Jansson & Ehnevid 1998).

C. A true combined endo–perio lesion refers to lesions originating from both endodontic and periodontal pathogens. They may occur concomitantly or independently. When lesions with different origins are coalesced, clinically it is very challenging to distinguish from other types of endo-perio lesions, such as primary endodontic lesion with secondary periodontal involvement.

D. The following examinations help the differential diagnosis between endodontic and periodontal disease (Silverstein et al. 1998).
a. *Vitality test*: In endodontic disease, the tooth is non-vital if pulp becomes necrotic; in periodontal disease, the tooth is vital in most cases.
b. *Plaque / calculus*: In endodontic disease, plaque or calculus may present, but they are not the primary cause of the disease; in periodontal disease, plaque or calculus is the primary cause.
c. *Pocket/probing depth*: In endodontic disease, a single and narrow pocket may present; in periodontal disease, generalized periodontal pockets may present and they are located relatively wide and coronally.
d. *Radiographics*: bone loss in endodontic disease is localized and mostly in the apical area; in periodontal disease, bone resorption is more generalized and mostly seen at the crestal bone.

E. If the conventional treatment is insufficient, alternative treatments should be considered. These alternatives include root resection/amputation (removal of the affected root); and regenerative techniques such as guided tissue regeneration and guided bone regeneration (Duggins et al. 1994; Green 1986).

References

Blomlof, L., Lengheden, A. & Linskog, S. (1992) Endodontic infection and calcium hydroxide treatment effects on periodontal healing in mature and immature replanted monkey teeth. *Journal of Clinical Periodontology* **29**, 652–658.

Duggins, I., Clay, J., Himel, V. et al. (1994) A combined endodontic retrofill and periodontal guided tissue regeneration for the repair of molar endodontic furcation perforations: report of a case. *Quintessence International* **25**, 109–114.

Green, E. N. (1986) Hemisection and root amputation. *Journal of the American Dental Association* **112**, 511–518.

Jansson, L. E. & Ehnevid, H. (1998) The influence of endodontic infection on periodontal status in mandibular molars. *Journal of Periodontology* **69**, 1392–1396.

Seltzer, S., Bender, I. B. & Ziontz, M. (1963) The interrelationship of pulp and periodontal disease. *Oral Surgery, Oral Medicine, Oral Pathology* **16**, 1474–1490.

Silverstein, L., Shatz, P. C., Amato, A. L. et al. (1998) A guide to diagnosing and treating endodontic and periodontal lesions. *Dentistry Today* **17**, 112–115.

Withers, J., Brunsvold, M., Killoy, W. et al. (1981) The relationship of palatogingival grooves to localized periodontal disease. *Journal of Periodontology* **52**, 41–44.

23

Traumatic Injuries:
Avulsed and Root-Fractured Maxillary Central Incisor

Bill Kahler and Louis M. Lin

LEARNING OBJECTIVES
- To understand how to provide appropriate emergency care immediately following dental trauma, including diagnosis and treatment.
- To understand how to use the American Association of Endodontists (AAE) guidelines as a guide in the management of dental trauma.

- To understand how to manage appropriately a tooth with horizontal root fracture when the pulp becomes necrotic and/or infected.
- To understand the importance of long-term follow-up of teeth in the area of trauma.

	Molars			Premolars		Canine	Incisors				Canine	Premolars		Molars		
							Maxillary arch									
Universal tooth designation system	1	2	3	4	5	6	7	8	9	10	11	12	13	14	15	16
International standards organization designation system	18	17	16	15	14	13	12	11	21	22	23	24	25	26	27	28
Palmer method	8⌐	7⌐	6⌐	5⌐	4⌐	3⌐	2⌐	1⌐	⌐1	⌐2	⌐3	⌐4	⌐5	⌐6	⌐7	⌐8

	Molars			Premolars		Canine	Incisors				Canine	Premolars		Molars		
Palmer method	8⌐	7⌐	6⌐	5⌐	4⌐	3⌐	2⌐	1⌐	⌐1	⌐2	⌐3	⌐4	⌐5	⌐6	⌐7	⌐8
International standards organization designation system	48	47	46	45	44	43	42	41	31	32	33	34	35	36	37	38
Universal tooth designation system	32	31	30	29	28	27	26	25	24	23	22	21	20	19	18	17
							Mandibular arch									
	Right									**Left**						

Clinical Cases in Endodontics, First Edition. Edited by Takashi Komabayashi.
© 2018 John Wiley & Sons, Inc. Published 2018 by John Wiley & Sons, Inc.

Chief Complaint

"The splint had come loose" on a tooth that had been root fractured and the avulsed coronal fragment came off.

Medical History

The patient (Pt) was a 10-year-old healthy male. Pt was taking no medication. Medical history was non-contributory.

The Pt was American Society of Anesthesiologists Physical Status Scale (ASA) Class I.

Dental History

The boy had fallen running down the stairs at home, which caused a horizontal mid-root fracture of tooth #8. The coronal fragment was avulsed and immediately placed in milk and re-implanted into the socket 1 hour later in the Emergency Department of a hospital. Tooth #8 was stabilized by interproximal composite resin. The periapical (PA) radiograph showed the socket of avulsed coronal fragment (Figure 23.1) and repositioned coronal fragment in the socket (Figure 23.2). A silk suture was placed for a gingival laceration. The splint de-bonded later that day and a composite resin and light wire splint was placed. The second splint de-bonded again and the Pt was referred to a specialist for management and seen the next day.

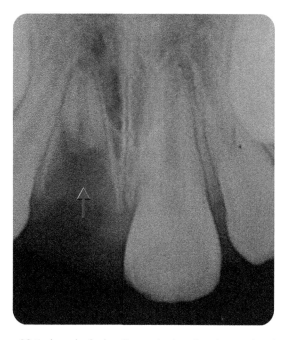

Figure 23.1 A periapical radiograph showing the retained apical fragment of the root of tooth #8 and the space (red arrow) from which the coronal fragment of the root was avulsed. The retained apical fragment has an open apex.

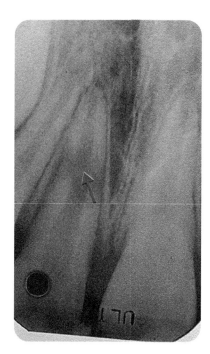

Figure 23.2 The coronal fragment of the root of tooth #8 was repositioned by the emergency dentist of a hospital and splinted with interproximal composite resin to teeth #7 and #9. The root fragments have been placed in close apposition (red arrow).

Clinical Evaluation (Diagnostic Procedures)
Examinations
Extra-oral Examination (EOE)

There was no asymmetry, swelling, or discoloration of the face. No palpable lymph nodes in neck area were present. Some swelling of the upper lip was noted.

Intra-oral Examination (IOE)

Oral hygiene was good. At the emergency clinic, a 4-0 silk suture had been placed for a gingival laceration. There was no swelling or draining sinus tract. A composite and wire splint had de-bonded from tooth #7. Interproximal composite resin between teeth #8 and #9 from the first splint was still present (Figure 23.3). Tooth #8 had grade 2 mobility. Tooth #9 had an uncomplicated crown fracture.

Diagnostic Tests

Tooth	#7	#8	#9	#10
Percussion	–	+	–	–
Palpation	–	+	–	–
Cold	+	–	+	+
EPT	Vague	–	+	Vague

EPT: Electric pulp test; +: Response to percussion or palpation, and normal response to cold and EPT; –: No response to percussions, palpation, cold, or EPT

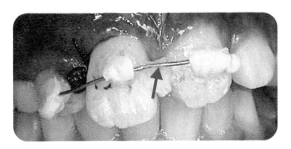

Figure 23.3 A clinical photograph of the second splint consisting of composite resin and light wire placed after failure of the interproximal composite resin splint. The remains of the first splint placed earlier that same day are seen between teeth #8 and #9 (red arrow). A 4/0 silk suture was placed between teeth #7 and #8 to unite a gingival laceration.

Radiographic Findings

Figure 23.1 shows a mid-root horizontal root fracture of tooth #8 where the coronal fragment of the root was avulsed. The retained apical fragment has an open apex. Figure 23.2 shows the repositioned coronal fragment.

Pretreatment Diagnosis
Pulpal

Pulp Necrosis, tooth #8

Apical

Normal Apical Tissues, tooth #8

Treatment Plan
Recommended

Emergency: Place a flexible splint
Definitive: Close follow-up of tooth #8

Alternative

If symptoms/signs of infection of tooth #8 develop, endodontic treatment of the coronal fragment will be performed.

Restorative

Composite resin

Prognosis

Favorable	Questionable	Unfavorable
	X	

Clinical Procedures: Treatment Record

First visit (Day 1): The prior splints of composite resin and wire were removed. The silk suture was also removed. A composite and Ribbond® fiber splint

(Ribbond, Seattle, WA, USA) was placed (Figure 23.4). A PA radiograph was taken to check the correct repositioning of the coronal fragment (Figure 23.5).

Second visit (1 week): One week review showed healing of the gingival tissue. Tooth #8 was asymptomatic (ASX).

Third visit (2 weeks): Again the tooth was ASX after another one week review.

Fourth visit (1 month): A gingival swelling was noted in the buccal (B) gingiva of tooth #8. Tooth #8 was extruded (Figure 23.6). A PA radiograph of tooth #8 revealed a space between the fractured fragments as well as loss of PA bone (Figure 23.7). The tooth did not respond to electric pulp test. A diagnosis of pulp necrosis and gingival abscess was made. The procedure and prognosis for root canal treatment of the coronal fragment was discussed with the Pt's parents, and informed consent was obtained. Tooth #8 was

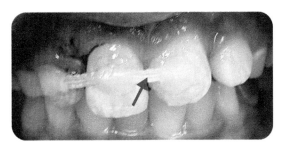

Figure 23.4 A clinical photograph of the third splint of composite resin and Ribbond® (red arrow) placed after the patient had been referred for specialist management.

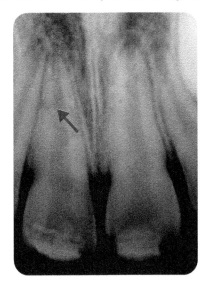

Figure 23.5 A periapical radiograph showing good apposition of the fractured root fragments with the third splint (red arrow).

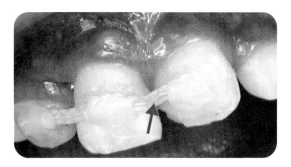

Figure 23.6 A clinical photograph taken 1 month after the initial injury showing the Ribbond® splint distended (red arrow) and tooth #8 extruded below the occlusal plane. There is a gingival swelling adjacent tooth #8.

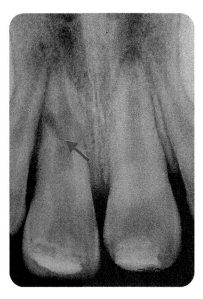

Figure 23.7 A periapical radiograph taken 1 month after the initial injury showing separation of the two fractured fragments (red arrow). Loss of alveolar bone on the distal aspect of tooth #8 is evident.

anesthetized with 1.8 cc, 2% lidocaine (lido) containing 1:100,000 epinephrine (epi) administered by local infiltration. A rubber dam (RD) was placed on tooth using a cuff technique with Wedjets® (Coltene, Altstätten, Switzerland). The length of the coronal fragment from the incisal edge to the level of fracture was determined radiographically with a size #40 Hedstrom file. The working length was 12 mm. The pulp chamber was accessed and necrotic tissue was removed with minimal mechanical debridement. The canal of the coronal fragment was irrigated with 1% sodium hypochlorite (NaOCl) solution, dried and dressed with $(Ca(OH)_2)$ to a level of 12 mm below the incisal edge. The access cavity was closed with Cavit™ (3M, Two Harbors, MN, USA) and glass ionomer cement, Fuji IX GP® (GC Corporation, Tokyo, Japan).

Fifth visit (3 months): The Pt was symptom free and the gingival tissue appeared healthy. A RD was placed on tooth #8 without local anesthesia. The tooth was accessed and irrigated with 1% NaOCl, and rinsed with 17% Ethylenediaminetetraacetic acid (EDTA). The canal was dried, and mineral trioxide aggregate (ProRoot® MTA; Dentsply Sirona, Johnson City, TN, USA) was placed in the canal using Buchanan pluggers to the level of fracture site. A wet cotton pellet was placed on the MTA to facilitate the setting of the material. The access cavity was restored with Cavit™ and glass ionomer cement. The fiber and composite resin splint was removed. The tooth had grade 1 mobility.

Sixth visit (3 months and 1 week): The tooth was isolated with a RD without local anesthesia. The access cavity was reopened and the cotton pellet removed. The setting of MTA was checked with an endodontic explorer. The access cavity was restored with composite resin. The coronal fragment was slightly displaced from the apical fragment (Figure 23.8).

Post-Treatment Evaluation

Seventh visit (1-year follow-up): Tooth #8 was ASX and had grade 1 mobility. A PA radiograph revealed blunting of the fractured fragments on the lateral borders of the root. Deposition of calcified material adjacent to the MTA and intracanal calcification of the apical fragment was evident. The coronal fragment was slightly displaced from the apical fragment. There was evidence of healing

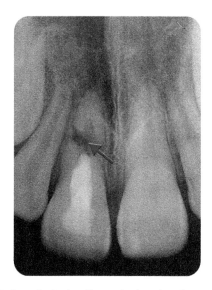

Figure 23.8 A periapical radiograph showing the coronal root fragment of tooth #8 root filled with MTA. The access cavity has been restored with glass ionomer cement and composite resin. The root fragments remain separated (red arrow).

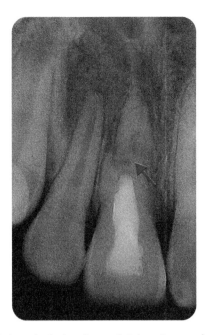

Figure 23.9 A periapical radiograph taken 1 year after the injury showing healing by deposition of calcific tissue between the fractured root fragments (red arrow). Intra-canal calcification of the apical fragment is evident. An incidental finding was the PA radiolucency associated with #7 consistent with a diagnosis of asymptomatic apical periodontitis (AAP). This tooth was responsive to cold pulp sensibility testing consistent with a false positive test. The management of this tooth is not discussed in this report.

of fractured fragments by interposition of calcific tissue. No inflammatory or replacement root resorption was noted. A large periapical radiolucency was associated with tooth #7 (Figure 23.9).

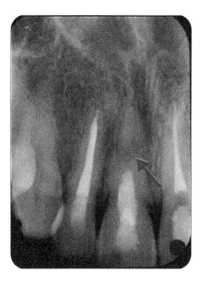

Figure 23.10 A periapical radiograph taken 10 years after the injury. Healing by hard tissue is likely as no periodontal ligament (PDL) space is evident between the previously fractured root fragments (red arrow). Further calcification of the apical fragment has occurred. Teeth #7 and #9 have been root filled. A favorable healing outcome, as evidenced by osseous repair for all root-filled teeth.

Eighth visit (10-year follow-up): Tooth #8 was ASX and had grade 1 mobility. A PA radiograph of tooth #8 showed similar presentation as observed ten years before. Teeth #7 and #9 were subsequently treated with non-surgical root canal therapy (NSRCT) because of development of pulpal–periapical disease (Figure 23.10).

Self-Study Questions

A. What are the appropriate tests to ensure an adequate diagnosis following dental trauma?

B. What are the important clinical parameters for outcomes for root-fractured teeth?

C. What are the important clinical parameters for outcomes for avulsed teeth?

D. What are the requirements for splinting of traumatized teeth?

E. Endodontic management for infected root-fractured teeth traditionally used long-term calcium hydroxide ($Ca(OH)_2$). What are the advantages/disadvantages of using mineral trioxide aggregate (MTA)?

Answers to Self-Study Questions

A. Clinical examination techniques for assessing the extent of injury to traumatized teeth include mobility testing, percussion sound, tenderness to percussion, and response to pulp testing. However, all these tests require clinical interpretation. For instance, mobility testing is not always clear as in the case of a luxation injury where the apex of the root may be locked in bone. A positive response to tenderness to percussion at the time of injury implies damage to the periodontal ligament and/or supporting structures. In contrast, persistent tenderness to percussion in the follow-up period is usually related to pulp necrosis and infection. Furthermore, the assessment of pulp vitality following dental trauma is an important diagnostic challenge as temporary loss of sensibility often occurs following traumatic injuries to the teeth. For instance, pulpal edema can cause loss of sensibility as well as torn or severed neurovascular supply to the pulp. A non-response to pulp sensibility testing also has prognostic significance in the follow-up period. For example, a non-response to pulp sensibility may have prognostic significance, in relation to pulp canal obliteration after luxation injuries, tissue union following root fractures, and pulp necrosis in combined crown fracture luxation injuries. Even color changes in the crown are reversible over time and are not suggestive of pulp necrosis. Therefore, judicious clinical judgement is required in diagnosis following dental trauma. Photographic documentation is also important for complete trauma assessment and may be required for later treatment planning, research, or legal claims (Andreasen & Kahler 2015a).

All initial examinations should include a radiographic assessment. Important parameters include the stage of root development, injuries to the root and supporting structures, and any displacement of the teeth. It is recommended that radiographic assessment include three different angulations and a steep occlusal view. The use of cone beam-computed tomography (CBCT) imaging has further enhanced trauma diagnosis, though generally CBCT should only be used when standard radiographic examination is unclear (Sigurdsson 2014; Andreasen

& Kahler 2015a). For instance, in this case presentation, conventional radiographic techniques clearly diagnosed the avulsion and root fracture of tooth #8, obviating the need for CBCT imaging.

Radiographic observations indicating pulp necrosis and infection following root fracture include widening or a diffusely outlined periodontal space, a radiolucency adjacent to the root fracture, and external inflammatory root resorption usually apparent 2–8 weeks following the injury (Andreasen & Kahler 2015b). In traumatized teeth, even if the pulp is completely devitalized, no radiographic periapical lesion will develop unless the pulp becomes infected. However, traumatized teeth sometimes show radiographic transient apical breakdown, not due to pulpal infection (Andreasen 1986).

A clinician should therefore consider the patient's presenting signs and symptoms, clinical test results and the radiographic assessments before deciding on any endodontic intervention. Often emergency care and further review may be all the treatment required. The aim of treating dental trauma is either to maintain or regain pulp vitality in traumatized teeth if possible (Sigurdsson 2014). However, this case report also highlights the importance of long-term follow-up, as the adjacent teeth, which were seemingly unaffected at the time of injury, subsequently required endodontic management.

B. In 2004, two landmark studies (Andreasen *et al.* 2004a, 2004b) of 400 root fractured teeth, showed 30% of teeth healed by hard tissue union of the fractured fragments, 5% healed with interposition of bone and connective tissue, 43% healed with interposition of connective tissue only, while only 22% showed non-healing as a result of pulp necrosis and infection (Andreasen *et al.* 2004a). A young age, immature root formation, minimal mobility, positive pulp sensibility testing, and optimal positioning of the fractured fragments were positively associated with pulpal and hard tissue repair. Healing was progressively worsened with increased diastasis between the fragments. In these studies, the highest frequency of healing was associated with fiberglass splints

CLINICAL CASES IN ENDODONTICS

(Andreasen *et al.* 2004b). Hence, as this case treatment was commenced in 2005, a fiberglass splint was employed. Unfortunately pulp necrosis and infection developed in this case and may have been due to the avulsion of the coronal fragment as discussed below.

C. Many studies have reported higher failure rates for avulsed teeth with open apices when compared to mature teeth. In a study of 400 replanted teeth where revascularization was considered possible, only 34% subsequently showed this favorable healing outcome (Andreasen *et al.* 1995a). Pulp necrosis was generally evident after just three weeks. If revascularization did occur, pulp sensibility changes were usually noted at six months and often associated with signs of pulp canal obliteration (Andreasen *et al.* 1995b). In the presented case, a fractured root is similar to an open apex scenario, so the risk of pulp necrosis was higher. However, timely endodontic management prevented the common sequelae of inflammatory replacement resorption. The risk of cell death to the periodontal ligament cells and subsequent replacement resorption is related to increased extra-alveolar storage time (Andreasen *et al.* 1995c). However, storage in milk for up to 3 hours has been shown to preserve the vitality of the periodontal ligament cells after extraction in an animal model (Blomlöf *et al.* 1980). Therefore, immediate replantation is recommended. In this case replacement resorption was avoided.

D. The AAE guidelines for the treatment of traumatized teeth recommend that root fractured teeth should be splinted for four weeks. In contrast, an avulsed tooth should only be splinted for two weeks (Sigurdsson 2014). Clinical judgement was required in this rare concomitant injury of a root fracture and avulsion injury. A flexible splint is considered important for favorable healing of the periodontal ligament and less incidence of ankylosis and replacement resorption, presumably due to physiological stimulation at a cellular level (Kahler & Heithersay 2008). However, in high cervical root fractures a more rigid split with a longer splinting duration of four months is recommended (Sigurdsson 2014). Many studies have shown that the type of splint and splinting duration are not significant variables on either pulpal or periodontal

outcomes following trauma to the teeth (Andreasen *et al.* 1995b, 1995c; Andreasen *et al.* 2004b). In this case, a flexible splint was placed for three months as there had been significant bone loss along the lateral border of the tooth, and the family was away for two months for school holidays. The removal of composite resin is usually associated with some iatrogenic damage to the enamel. Recently, a new splinting regime has been advocated with resin activated glass-ionomer cement suitable for orthodontic bracket cementation which has allowed the development of an alternative simplified splinting regimen for traumatized teeth, providing ease of application and removal with minimal or no iatrogenic to enamel (Kahler *et al.* 2016).

E. Pulp necrosis and infection following root fracture is usually limited to the coronal fragment. When the root canal is wide in immature teeth or mid-root fractures, there are difficulties in achieving adequate obturation with gutta-percha. Traditionally this has required the use of long-term dressing with calcium hydroxide to create a hard tissue barrier at the fracture site, which then allows for a root filling to be placed. This procedure has been shown to have successful long-term outcomes. However, the apical barrier is often irregular and consists of a cementum-like calcific material that includes areas of soft connective tissue, and the procedure requires long-term dressing with calcium hydroxide which may weaken the root. Furthermore, multiple appointments may be required before an adequate apical barrier is formed (Cvek 2007).

Mineral trioxide aggregate (MTA) placed at the level of the fracture site is an alternative to calcium hydroxide. MTA has excellent anti-bacterial and osseo-inductive properties. Histological studies have demonstrated a more homogenous calcific barrier for MTA barrier technique when compared to teeth treated with calcium hydroxide. MTA is resistant to microbial leakage due to its adaption to the root canal walls and penetration into the dentinal tubules (Parirokh & Torabinejad 2010). MTA also does not appear to weaken teeth as has been proposed for calcium hydroxide (Andreasen, Munksgaard & Bakland 2006). A number of case reports have shown good long-term outcomes where MTA has been used. This case shows a successful 10-year outcome.

References

Andreasen, F. M. (1986) Transient apical breakdown and its relation to color and sensibility changes after luxation injuries to teeth. *Dental Traumatology* **2**, 9–19.

Andreasen, F. M. & Kahler, B. (2015a) Diagnosis of acute dental trauma: The importance of standardized documentation: A review. *Dental Traumatology* **31**, 340–349.

Andreasen, F. M. & Kahler, B. (2015b) Pulpal response after acute dental injury in the permanent dentition: Clinical implications: A review. *Journal of Endodontics* **41**, 299–308.

Andreasen, J. O., Borum, M. K., Jacobsen, H. L. *et al.* (1995a) Replantation of 400 avulsed permanent incisors. 1. Diagnosis of healing complications. *Endodontics and Dental Traumatology* **11**, 51–58.

Andreasen, J. O., Borum, M. K., Jacobsen, H. L. *et al.* (1995b) Replantation of 400 avulsed permanent incisors. 2. Factors related to pulpal healing. *Endodontics and Dental Traumatology* **11**, 59–68.

Andreasen, J. O., Borum, M. K., Jacobsen, H. L. *et al.* (1995c) Replantation of 400 avulsed permanent incisors. 4. Factors related to periodontal ligament healing. *Endodontics and Dental Traumatology* **11**, 76–89.

Andreasen, J. O., Andreasen, F. M., Mejare, I. *et al.* (2004a) Healing of 400 intra-alveolar root fractures. 1. Effect of pre-injury and injury factors such as sex, age, stage of root development, fracture type, location of fracture and severity of dislocation. *Dental Traumatology* **20**, 192–202.

Andreasen, J. O., Andreasen, F. M., Mejare, I. *et al.* (2004b) Healing of 400 intra-alveolar root fractures. 2. Effect of treatment factors such as treatment delay, repositioning, splinting type and period and antibiotics. *Dental Traumatology* **20**, 203–211.

Andreasen, J. O., Munksgaard, E. C. & Bakland, L. K. (2006) Comparison of fracture resistance in root canals of immature sheep teeth after filling with calcium hydroxide or MTA. *Dental Traumatology* **22**, 154–156.

Blomlöf, L., Lindskog, D., Hedstrom, K. G. *et al.* (1980) Vitality of periodontal ligament cells after storage of monkey teeth in milk or saliva. *Scandinavian Journal of Dental Research* **88**, 441–445.

Cvek, M. (2007) Endodontic management and the use of calcium hydroxide in traumatized permanent teeth. In: *Textbook and Color Atlas of Traumatic Injuries to the Teeth* (eds. J. O. Andreasen, F. M. Andreasen & L. Andersson) 4th edn, pp. 598–657. Oxford: Blackwell.

Kahler, B. & Heithersay, G. S. (2008) An evidence-based appraisal of splinting luxated, avulsed and root-fractured teeth. *Dental Traumatology* **24**, 2–10.

Kahler, B., Hu, J. Y., Marriot-Smith, C. S. *et al.* (2016) Splinting of teeth following trauma: A review and a new splinting recommendation. *Australian Dental Journal* **61**, (Suppl. 1), 59–73.

Parirokh, M. & Torabinejad, M. (2010) Mineral trioxide aggregate: A comprehensive literature review. Part III: Clinical applications, drawbacks, and mechanism of action. *Journal of Endodontics* **36**, 400–413.

Sigurdsson, A. (2014) The treatment of dental traumatic injuries. *Endodontics: Colleagues for Excellence Newsletter.* Chicago: American Association of Endodontists.

24

Incompletely Developed Apices

Nathaniel T. Nicholson

LEARNING OBJECTIVES

- To understand the procedures of apexogenesis, apexification, apical barrier technique, and revascularization.
- To understand when to utilize these procedures in managing incompletely developed apices.
- To understand the clinical steps and materials for a regeneration procedure.
- To understand the clinical steps and materials for apexogenesis.
- To understand the clinical steps and materials for apical barrier technique.
- To understand the importance of maintaining pulp vitality.

	Molars			Premolars		Canine	Incisors				Canine	Premolars		Molars		
							Maxillary arch									
Universal tooth designation system	1	2	3	4	5	6	7	8	9	10	11	12	13	14	15	16
International standards organization designation system	18	17	16	15	14	13	12	11	21	22	23	24	25	26	27	28
Palmer method	8⌋	7⌋	6⌋	5⌋	4⌋	3⌋	2⌋	1⌋	⌊1	⌊2	⌊3	⌊4	⌊5	⌊6	⌊7	⌊8
Palmer method	8⌉	7⌉	6⌉	5⌉	4⌉	3⌉	2⌉	1⌉	⌈1	⌈2	⌈3	⌈4	⌈5	⌈6	⌈7	⌈8
International standards organization designation system	48	47	46	45	44	43	42	41	31	32	33	34	35	36	37	38
Universal tooth designation system	32	31	30	29	28	27	26	25	24	23	22	21	20	19	18	17
							Mandibular arch									
		Right								**Left**						

Clinical Cases in Endodontics, First Edition. Edited by Takashi Komabayashi.
© 2018 John Wiley & Sons, Inc. Published 2018 by John Wiley & Sons, Inc.

Chief Complaint

"My dentist said I needed to come see you."

Medical History

The patient (Pt) was a 12-year-old male. Vital signs were as follows: blood pressure (BP) 112/76 mmHg; pulse 76 beats per minute (BPM). He had no known drug allergies (NKDA), no medical conditions and did not take any medication.

The Pt was American Society of Anesthesiologists Physical Status Scale (ASA) Class I.

Dental History

The Pt had a history of routine dental care with the general dentist. He had never had any decay or any other oral problems. Pt was asymptomatic and receiving orthodontic treatment with bands and wires. The orthodontist recommended trying to save tooth #31, because the orthodontist did not think he could move tooth #32 into the position of tooth #31. Pt was then treated by a periodontist for gingivectomy of tooth #31 to allow access to treat. Pt was subsequently referred for treatment of tooth #31.

Clinical Evaluation (Diagnostic Procedures)
Examinations
Extra-oral Examination (EOE)

No swelling or lymphadenopathy was found. The temporomandibular joint showed no popping/clicking or deviation.

Intra-oral Examination (IOE)

There was no swelling, oral cancer screening was within normal limits (WNL) and no pathosis was detected. Tooth #31 appeared intact, except for a small explorer stick on occlusal surface. Teeth #19 and #30 had orthodontic bands with wire running around the arch with brackets on the anterior teeth. Teeth #28 and #29 were unrestored. Tooth #30 also appeared unrestored.

Diagnostic Tests

Tooth	#29	#30	#31
Percussion	–	–	–
Palpation	–	–	–
Endo Ice®	+	+	+
Probing	2–3 mm	2–3 mm	2–3 mm
Mobility	–	–	–

+: Response to percussion or palpation, and normal response to Endo Ice®;
-: No response to percussion or palpation, no mobility

Radiographic Findings

Although it was extremely difficult to get a radiograph of the tooth, tooth #31 had a large coronal radiolucency encroaching on the pulp chamber (Figure 24.2). There appeared to be normal root development on tooth #31, but root apices were still open (Figure 24.1). Tooth #30 appeared normal. Tooth #32 crown was partially visible. No other pathosis was observed on periapical (PA) radiograph.

Pretreatment Diagnosis
Pulpal

Asymptomatic Irreversible Pulpitis, tooth #31

Apical

Normal Apical Tissues, tooth #31

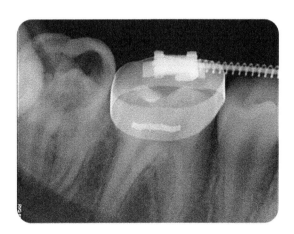

Figure 24.1 Preoperative periapical radiograph of tooth #31 showing incompletely developed apices.

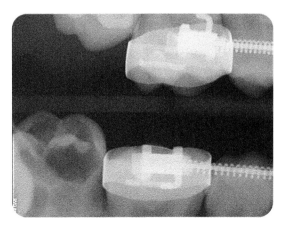

Figure 24.2 Preoperative bitewing radiograph showing the extensive coronal radiolucency encroaching on the pulp.

Treatment Plan

Recommended

Emergency: None
Definitive: Pulpotomy for apexogenesis

Alternative

No treatment; Apexification; Direct Pulp Cap; Indirect Pulp Cap; Extraction

Restorative

Coronal Restoration with resin or amalgam, Crown

Prognosis

Favorable	Questionable	Unfavorable
X		

Clinical Procedures: Treatment Record

First visit (Day 1): The medical history, vitals recorded, clinical and radiographic evaluation completed were reviewed with grandmother, as were findings, options, risks, benefits, and alternatives. Grandmother elected pulpotomy for apexogenesis on tooth #31 and informed consent was obtained. Benzocaine 20% topical was applied, and 144 mg of 4% articaine with 0.018 mg of epinephrine (epi) (1:200,000) was administered via inferior alveolar nerve block and long buccal nerve blocks. Rubber dam isolation (RDI) was used (Figure 24.3) with OpalDam® (Ultradent, South Jordan, UT, USA) around tooth and clamp. The occlusal of the tooth was opened, and while removing decay, the pulp was exposed (Figure 24.4). All decay was then removed, which resulted in the clamp coming off the tooth. An orthodontic band was fitted and cemented with Ketac™ (3M, Two Harbors, MN, USA) cement (Figure 24.5) after placing a sterile cotton ball over the pulp. The pulp

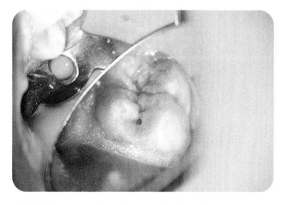

Figure 24.3 Preoperative photograph showing intact occlusal surface.

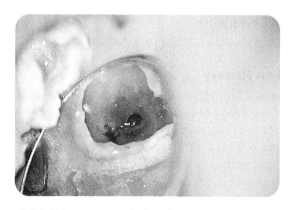

Figure 24.4 Pulp exposure during decay removal.

chamber was accessed and the cotton pellet was removed. The coronal pulp tissue was removed with a high-speed diamond with water spray. Hemostasis was obtained (Figure 24.6) with a 2.5% sodium hypochlorite (NaOCl)-saturated cotton pellet after a few minutes and white mineral trioxide aggregate (White ProRoot® MTA; Dentsply Sirona, Johnson City, TN, USA) was placed in the pulp chamber (Figure 24.7). The tooth was then temporized with Fuji Triage® glass ionomer (GC America Inc., Alsip, IL, USA). The RDI was removed, occlusion was checked, a postoperative radiograph (Figure 24.8) was exposed, postoperative instructions were given, the need for coronal restoration was stressed, and the Pt was dismissed in good condition.

Post-Treatment Evaluation

Second visit (1 year 1 month follow-up): Clinical and radiographic exams were completed. PA of tooth #31

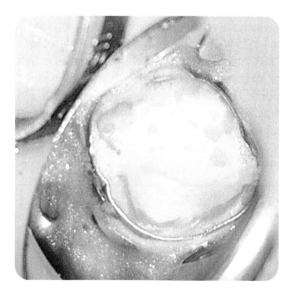

Figure 24.5 Orthodontic band cemented on with Ketac™ cement (rubber dam clamp popped off and building up tooth was necessary in order to reapply clamp).

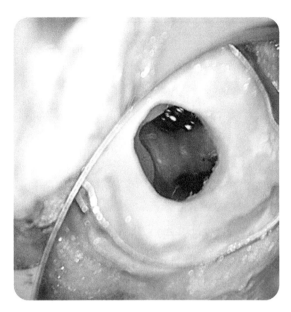

Figure 24.6 Pulp hemostasis after pulpotomy and decay removal completed.

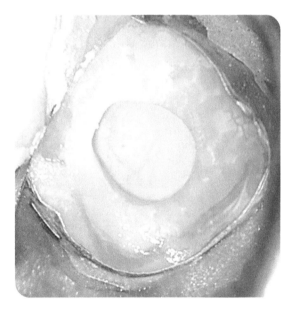

Figure 24.7 MTA placed in pulp chamber.

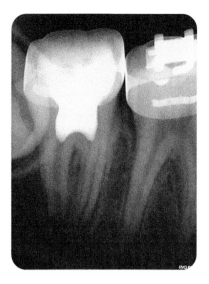

Figure 24.8 Postoperative radiograph (taken with sensor vertical).

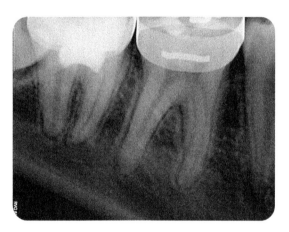

Figure 24.9 Follow-up 1 year 1 month.

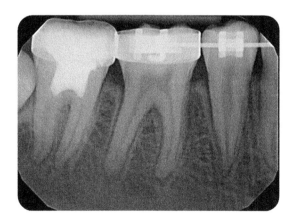

Figure 24.10 Follow-up 1 year 9 months.

(Figure 24.9) showed continued root development. The Pt remained asymptomatic; there were no signs of pathosis, but tooth #31 still had a temporary filling. The importance of having the tooth restored was stressed.

Third visit (1 year 9 month follow-up): Clinical and radiographic exams were completed. PA of tooth #31 (Figure 24.10) showed continued root development. The Pt remained asymptomatic, with no signs of pathosis, but tooth #31 still had temporary filling. The importance of having the tooth restored was stressed.

Fourth visit (2 year 3 month follow-up): Clinical and radiographic exams were completed. PA of tooth #31 (Figure 24.11) showed root development complete. Pt

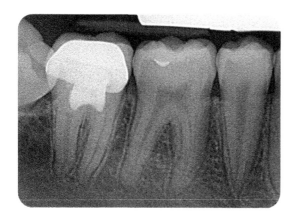

Figure 24.11 Follow-up 2 years 3 months.

remained asymptomatic, with no signs of pathosis, and tooth had been restored with a porcelain-fused-to-metal crown with margins that were within normal limits (WNL).

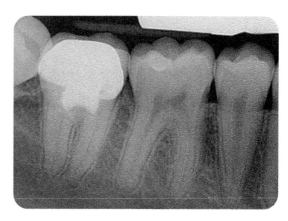

Figure 24.12 Follow-up 3 years 7 months.

Fifth visit (3 year 7 month follow-up): Clinical and radiographic exams were completed. PA of tooth #31 (Figure 24.12) showed apices still appearing normal. Pt remained asymptomatic, with no signs of pathosis, and margins of crown were WNL.

Self-Study Questions

A. What are the treatment options for teeth with incompletely developed apices with a pulpal diagnosis of necrotic pulp? Define each option.

B. What are the treatment options for teeth with incompletely developed apices with a pulpal diagnosis of normal pulp, reversible pulpitis, or irreversible pulpitis?

C. Describe the clinical steps for a regeneration procedure.

D. Describe the clinical steps for an apexogenesis procedure.

E. Describe the clinical steps for an apical barrier technique.

Answers to Self-Study Questions

A. With incompletely developed apices with a necrotic pulp, the treatment options are apexification, apical barrier, or a regeneration procedure.

- **Apexification** is defined as "A method to induce a calcified barrier in a root with an open apex or the continued apical development of an incompletely formed root in teeth with necrotic pulps" (*AAE Glossary of Endodontic Terms* 2016). Apexification is completed in multiple visits during which calcium hydroxide is placed in the root canal to induce an apical barrier and checked each visit for a calcific apical barrier. One disadvantage of apexification is that it takes an average of 12.9 months (Dominguez Reyes, Muñoz & Aznar 2005), with time ranging from 5 to 20 months (Sheehy & Roberts 1997). Moreover, *in vitro* studies have shown calcium hydroxide decreases the fracture strength of immature teeth with prolonged use (Andreasen, Farik & Munksgaard 2002).

- **Apical barrier technique** is defined as "placement of a matrix in the apical region to prevent extrusion of endodontic filling material; typically refers to teeth with open apices" (*AAE Glossary of Endodontic Terms* 2016). This technique is completed in one or two visits, depending on whether the clinician wants to check if the barrier material has fully set prior to restoring the tooth. Mineral trioxide aggregate (MTA) (Torabinejad, Watson & Pitt Ford 1993) is commonly used, but many other calcium silicate materials, such as Biodentine® (Septodont, Lancaster, PA, USA) and EndoSequence® Root Repair Material (Brassler, Savannah, GA, USA), have come on the market since MTA was developed.

- **Pulpal regeneration technique** is defined as "biologically-based procedures designed to physiologically replace damaged tooth structures, including dentin and root structures, as well as cells of the pulp-dentin complex" (*AAE Glossary of Endodontic Terms* 2016). Basically, the pulp space is disinfected and pulpal-like tissue is encouraged to form inside the root to continue root development (i.e., more dentin to thicken the root and increase its length).

B. With incompletely developed apices with a pulpal diagnosis of normal pulp, reversible pulpitis, symptomatic irreversible pulpitis, or asymptomatic irreversible pulpitis, apexogenesis is the treatment of choice.

- Apexogenesis is defined as "[a] vital pulp therapy procedure performed to encourage continued physiological development and formation of the root end; frequently used to describe vital pulp therapy…" (*AAE Glossary of Endodontic Terms* 2016). The term includes direct pulp cap, indirect pulp cap, partial (Cvek) pulpotomy or pulpotomy. Direct pulp cap is where the exposed pulp is covered with MTA or any other calcium silicate material; historically calcium hydroxide was used. Indirect pulp cap means the pulp is never exposed clinically by leaving a layer of decay over the top of the pulp and covering with MTA or any other calcium silicate material, and the tooth is definitively restored, or the tooth is temporarily restored and re-entered at a later date to completely remove the remaining decay. Pulpotomy is where the coronal pulp tissue is partially (Cvek) removed or the coronal pulpal tissue is removed (complete pulpotomy), the pulp stump(s) is (are) covered with MTA or any other calcium silicate material, and the tooth is restored.

C. The clinical steps for Regeneration (adopted from the *AAE Clinical Considerations for a Regenerative Procedure*) are as follows:

First Appointment

- Obtain informed consent.
- Use a rubber dam to isolate tooth after local anesthesia administration.
- Access and irrigate with 20 ml per canal of 1.5% sodium hypochlorite (NaOCl; Martin *et al.* 2014) taking precaution to prevent irrigation extrusion (i.e., side vented needle or EndoVac® [Kerr, Orange, CA, USA]). Then irrigate 1 mm from the end of the root with 20 ml per canal of saline or Ethylenediaminetetraacetic acid (EDTA) over the course of 5 minutes.

- Dry canal(s) with paper points.
- Use a syringe to place calcium hydroxide paste (e.g., Ultracal XS® [Ultradent, South Jordan, UT, USA]) into the canal(s). Syringeable versions of calcium hydroxide are easier to remove at subsequent appointments than calcium hydroxide powder mixed with water.
- Alternatively, use triple antibiotic paste in a mix of 1:1:1 ciprofloxacin: metronidazole: minocycline to a final concentration of 0.1–1.0 mg/ml instead of calcium hydroxide. The minocycline in triple antibiotic paste has been shown to cause tooth discoloration, but sealing the pulp chamber with bonding agent and keeping paste below the cementoenamel junction (CEJ) can help prevent this complication, as can using double antibiotic paste (omitting the minocycline from the triple antibiotic paste).
- Temporize coronal access with material of choice (e.g., Cavit™ [3M, Two Harbors, MN, USA], Fuji Triage® [GC America Inc., Alsip, IL, USA] glass ionomer, etc.) at least 3–4 mm thick for proper seal.

Second Appointment (1–4 weeks later)

- Evaluate for the presence of infection, like swelling or sinus tract. If still present, consider using antimicrobial for longer or the use of a different antimicrobial (i.e., switch calcium hydroxide to triple antibiotic paste or vice versa).
- Use a rubber dam to isolate the tooth after local anesthesia administration with 3% mepivacaine (no epinephrine or other vasoconstrictor).
- Remove temporary restoration.
- Irrigate with about 20 ml per canal of 17% EDTA.
- Dry the canal(s) with paper points.
- Over-instrument into the periapical tissues (precurved endodontic file, endo explorer, etc.) to create bleeding into the canal space and allow blood to fill to level of CEJ. Some authors advocate using platelet-rich plasma, platelet rich fibrin or autologous fibrin matrix alternatively for creating a blood clot in the canal system.
- Place a resorbable collagen matrix (CollaPlug® [Zimmer Dental, Carlsbad, CA, USA], HeliPLUG® [Integra Miltex Plainsboro, NJ, USA], etc.) over the formed blot clot, if needed.
- Place ProRoot® MTA (Dentsply Sirona, Johnson City, TN, USA) white.

- Alternatively, in place of MTA, any other calcium silicate cement (e.g., Biodentine® and EndoSequence® Root Repair Material) can be used to prevent staining of the tooth.
- GC Fuji II® (GC America Inc., Alsip, IL, USA) glass ionomer is placed in a 3–4 mm layer over the MTA or other material used.
- Follow-up in 6 months, 1 year, and yearly thereafter.

D. The clinical steps for an apexogenesis procedure are as follows:
- Obtain informed consent.
- Use a rubber dam to isolate tooth after local anesthesia administration.
- Remove all decay, if present, and if pulp is exposed (Figure 24.13), obtain hemostasis with a 3–6% NaOCl-saturated cotton pellet placed over the pulp exposure (Figure 24.14).
- Note: If an indirect pulp cap is desired, leave a layer of decay over the top of the pulp, but ensure all circumferential margins are caries free. Then place MTA or any other calcium silicate material over the top of the decay, and restore the tooth either temporarily or definitively (Maltz *et al.* 2002).
- If after 10 minutes pulpal hemostasis is not obtained (Figure 24.15), perform a partial pulpomtomy by carefully removing a few millimeters of pulpal tissue with a diamond bur in a high-speed hand piece with copious water coolant. After another 5–10 minutes of using a 3–6% NaOCl-saturated cotton pellet, observe the pulp for bleeding. You may have

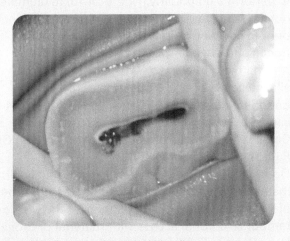

Figure 24.13 Preoperative pulpal bleeding.

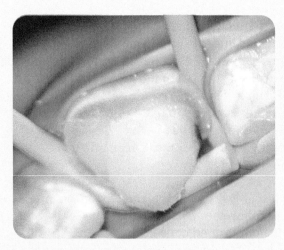

Figure 24.14 Sodium hypochlorite-saturated cotton pellet placed over pulp.

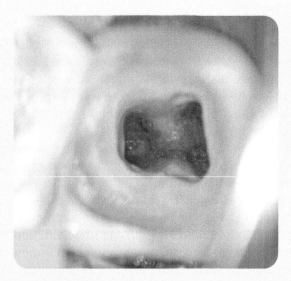

Figure 24.16 Pulpotomy on a molar.

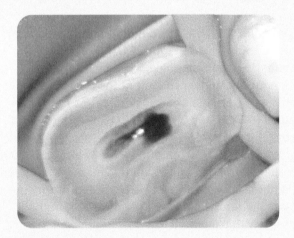

Figure 24.15 Pulp still bleeding after 10 minutes of use of sodium hypochlorite saturated cotton pellet.

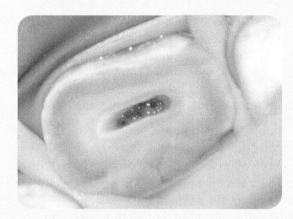

Figure 24.17 Pulp hemostasis after removing a few more millimeters of pulpal tissue and replacement of sodium hypochlorite pellet for a few minutes.

to perform a pulpotomy (Figure 24.16) to ultimately obtain hemostasis. Hemostasis must be obtained prior to covering pulp with MTA (Figure 24.17; Bogen and Chandler 2008).

• Alternatively, in place of MTA, any other calcium silicate cement (e.g., Biodentine® and EndoSequence® Root Repair Material; Figure 24.18) can be used to prevent staining of the tooth.

• Cover with a thin layer of glass ionomer (e.g., GC Fuji Lining™ LC; Figure 24.19).

• Optional (only if MTA is used, but not required): Instead of covering with a layer of glass ionomer, place a wet (water) cotton pellet over the MTA and temporize coronal access with material of choice (e.g., Cavit™, Fuji Triage® glass ionomer, etc.).

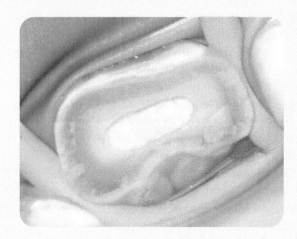

Figure 24.18 Endosequence® Root Repair Material covering pulp.

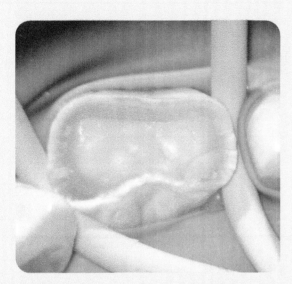

Figure 24.19 Glass ionomer placed to cover Endosequence® Root Repair Material (tooth ready to restore).

Bring patient back after at least 4 hours to check if MTA is initially set.
- Definitively restore the tooth.
- Follow-up in 6 months, 1 year, and yearly thereafter.

E. The clinical steps for the apical barrier technique are as follows:
- Obtain informed consent (see preoperative radiograph Figure 24.20).

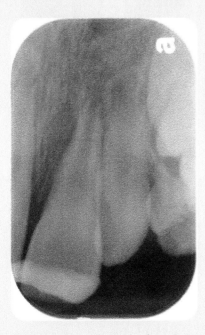

Figure 24.20 Preoperative radiograph of tooth #9 with open apex (history of avulsion, replanted, and splint).

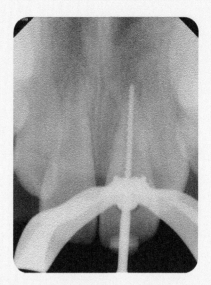

Figure 24.21 Working-length radiograph.

- Use a rubber dam to isolate tooth after local anesthesia administration.
- Remove all decay, if present.
- Access and obtain working length (Figure 24.21). Clean, shape, and disinfect the canal(s) with NaOCl irrigation after obtaining working length.
- Dry the canal(s) with paper points.
- Optional: Place calcium hydroxide paste (e.g., Ultracal XS®), temporize coronal access, and bring patient back within 1 month to prevent weakening the root from prolonged use of calcium hydroxide (Andreasen, Munksgaard, & Bakland 2006).
- Optional: Place a resorbable collagen matrix (CollaPlug, HeliPLUG, etc.) or calcium sulfate hemihydrate (e.g., Dentogen® [Orthogen, Springfield, NJ, USA]) into the periapical region until an apical stop is developed at working length. This prevents extrusion of material in the next step.
- Place 5 mm of MTA (Al-Kahtani *et al.* 2005) or any other calcium silicate cements (e.g. Biodentine® and Endosequence® Root Repair Material) in the apical portion of root. This material should extend to working length (Figure 24.22).
- Optional (only if MTA is used, but not required): Place a wet (water) cotton pellet over the MTA and temporize coronal access with material of choice (e.g., Cavit™, Fuji Triage® glass ionomer, etc.). Bring patient back after at least 4 hours to check if MTA is initially set.

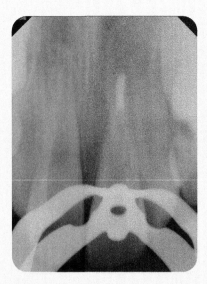

Figure 24.22 MTA apical barrier of about 5 mm.

- Place a layer of pulp canal sealer (e.g., AH Plus® [Dentsply Sirona]) and backfill with thermoplasticized gutta-percha (Figure 24.23) and restore definitively (Figure 24.24) or bond fiber post(s) in canal space and restore access definitively (Ree 2015).
- Follow-up in 6 months (Figure 24.25), 1 year (Figure 24.26), and yearly thereafter.

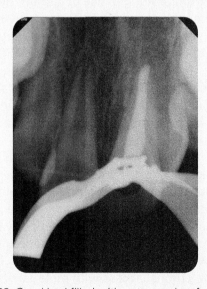

Figure 24.23 Canal backfilled with gutta-percha after coating canal with sealer.

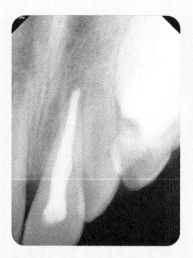

Figure 24.24 Access restored with composite resin.

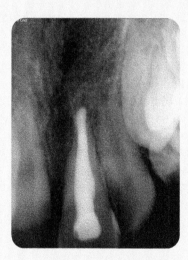

Figure 24.25 Follow-up 6 months.

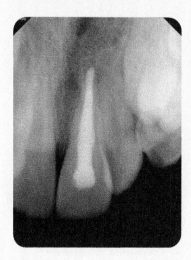

Figure 24.26 Follow-up 1 year.

References

Al-Kahtani, A., Shostad, S., Schifferle, R. *et al.* (2005) In-vitro evaluation of micro-leakage of an orthograde apical plug of mineral trioxide aggregate in permanent teeth with simulated immature apices. *Journal of Endodontics* **31**, 117–119.

American Association of Endodontists (2016) *AAE Clinical Considerations for a Regenerative Procedure* [Online]. Available: http://www.aae.org/uploadedfiles/publications_and_research/research/currentregenerativeendodonticconsiderations.pdf

American Association of Endodontists (2016) *Glossary of Endodontic Terms* [Online]. Available: http://www.nxtbook.com/nxtbooks/aae/endodonticglossary2016/.

Andreasen, J. O., Farik, B. & Munksgaard, E. C. (2002) Long-term calcium hydroxide as a root canal dressing may increase risk of root fracture. *Dental Traumatology* **18**, 134–137.

Andreasen, J. O., Munksgaard, E. C. & Bakland, L. K. (2006) Comparison of fracture resistance in root canals of immature sheep teeth after filling with calcium hydroxide or MTA. *Dental Traumatology* **22**, 154–156.

Bogen, G. & Chandler, N. P. (2008) Vital pulp therapy. In: *Ingle's Endodontics* (eds. J. I. Ingle, L. K. Bakland, & J. C. Baumgartner) 6th edn, p.1310. Hamilton, ON: BC Decker.

Dominguez, R. A., Muñoz, M. L. & Aznar, M. T. (2005) Study of calcium hydroxide apexification in 26 young permanent incisors. *Dental Traumatology* **21**, 141–145.

Maltz, M., de Oliveira, E. F., Fontanella, V. *et al.* (2002) A clinical, microbiologic, and radiographic study of deep caries lesions after incomplete caries removal. *Quintessence International* **33**, 151–159.

Martin, D. E., De Almeida, J. F., Henry, M. A. *et al.* (2014) Concentration-dependent effect of sodium hypochlorite on stem cells of apical papilla survival and differentiation. *Journal of Endodontics* **40**, 51–55.

Ree, M. (2015) Clinical management of teeth with open apices with the apical barrier technique. In: *Best Practices in Endodontics: A Desk Reference* (eds. R. S. Schwartz & V. Canakapalli), pp. 304–306. Chicago: Quintessence.

Sheehy, E. C. & Roberts, G. J. (1997) Use of calcium hydroxide for apical barrier formation and healing in non-vital immature permanent teeth: A review. *British Dental Journal* **183**, 241–246.

Torabinejad, M., Watson, T. F. & Pitt Ford, T. R. (1993) Sealing ability of a mineral trioxide aggregate when used as a root end filling material. *Journal of Endodontics* **19**, 591–595.

25

External/Internal Resorption

Keivan Zoufan, Takashi Komabayashi, and Qiang Zhu

LEARNING OBJECTIVES
- To understand the classifications of tooth resorption.
- To understand the etiology of tooth resorption.
- To understand the treatment of tooth resorption.

	Molars			Premolars		Canine	Incisors				Canine	Premolars		Molars		
							Maxillary arch									
Universal tooth designation system	1	2	3	4	5	6	7	8	9	10	11	12	13	14	15	16
International standards organization designation system	18	17	16	15	14	13	12	11	21	22	23	24	25	26	27	28
Palmer method	8|	7|	6|	5|	4|	3|	2|	1|	|1	|2	|3	|4	|5	|6	|7	|8
Palmer method	8|	7|	6|	5|	4|	3|	2|	1|	|1	|2	|3	|4	|5	|6	|7	|8
International standards organization designation system	48	47	46	45	44	43	42	41	31	32	33	34	35	36	37	38
Universal tooth designation system	32	31	30	29	28	27	26	25	24	23	22	21	20	19	18	17
							Mandibular arch									
	Right										**Left**					

Chief Complaint

"My tooth hurts when I drink or eat something cold. The pain lasts for several minutes. My dentist said I have a big cavity and the tooth may not be savable."

Medical History

The patient (Pt) was a 26-year-old male. Vital signs were as follows: Blood pressure (BP) 118/78 mmHg right arm seated; pulse 76 beats per minute (BPM) and regular; respiratory rate (RR) 18 breaths per minute. A complete review of systems revealed a history of sinus problems related to seasonal allergies. The Pt admitted to smoking one pack of cigarettes per day and had no known drug allergies (NKDA). He was taking 600 mg ibuprofen 4 times per day for dental pain.

The Pt was American Society of Anesthesiologists Physical Status Scale (ASA) Class I.

Dental History

Pt was referred for an evaluation and treatment (Tx) of tooth #23. Pt complained of sensitivity to cold from tooth #23. The previous week the sensitivity to cold got worse and the pain lasted longer. He contacted his general dentist who examined him a few hours prior and referred the Pt to the office. His oral hygiene was fair. He had a few restorations and moderate gingivitis. No history of orthodontic Tx or trauma.

Clinical Evaluation (Diagnostic Procedures)
Examinations
Extra-oral Examination (EOE)

Pt was alert, normally developed, and not stressed. The EOE revealed no swelling, no sinus tract, and no lymphadenopathy in the submandibular and neck areas.

Intra-oral Examination (IOE)

Soft tissue appeared normal. A pinkish discoloration and large cavitation were noted near the disto-buccal (DB) surface of tooth #23. A 4 mm probing defect was present along the DB line angle of tooth #23. No other resorptive lesion was noted clinically in any other teeth. All teeth had normal physiological mobility.

Diagnostic Tests

Tooth	#22	#23	#24
Percussion	–	–	–
Palpation	–	Tender in buccal gingiva	–
Endo Ice®	+	Lingering pain	+

+: Normal response to Endo Ice®; -: No response to percussion or palpation

Radiographic Findings

The periapical (PA) radiograph revealed a large irregular radiolucency on the distal (D) aspect of tooth #23 extending to the level of the crestal bone and into the root (Figure 25.1). Tooth #23 had Class 3 invasive cervical resorption. There was evidence of crest bone loss. No periapical radiolucency was noted for tooth #23. No other resorptive lesion was noted in other mandibular anterior teeth.

Pretreatment Diagnosis
Pulpal

Symptomatic Irreversible Pulpitis, tooth #23

Apical

Normal Apical Tissues, tooth #23

Treatment Plan
Recommended

Emergency: Pulpal Debridement and Surgical Repair
Definitive: Non-surgical Root Canal Therapy (NSRCT)

Alternative

Extraction; Orthodontic Extrusion and Non-surgical Approach

Restorative

Composite restoration followed by a full coverage restoration

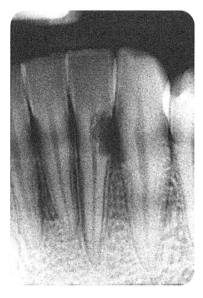

Figure 25.1 Preoperative radiograph reveals an irregular radiolucency extending both coronally and into the radicular tooth structure on the distal cervical side of tooth #23.

Prognosis

Favorable	Questionable	Unfavorable
	X	

Clinical Procedures: Treatment Record

First visit (Day 1): The medical history was reviewed (RMHX). Pt agreed to proceed with a periodontal flap and lesion excavation before finalizing the Tx plan. Consent was obtained. Local anesthesia was administered as follows: 108 mg 2% lidocaine (lido)/0.054 mg epinephrine (epi) (1:100.000). A full-thickness mucoperiopstal flap was reflected using sulcular incision from mesial (M) of tooth #20 to the D of tooth #27. A 6 x 8 mm resorptive defect was present on tooth #23 extending to the level of crestal bone. The lesion was excavated. It was friable and did not provide proper texture for a biopsy specimen. The tooth was then evaluated under microscope (Global Surgical Corporation, St. Louis, MO, USA). The tooth structure was solid beneath the defect. Trichloracetic acid (CCl$_3$COOH; Sigma-Aldrich, St. Louis, MO, USA) was applied by a small cotton pellet on the resorptive lesion for 4 minutes and rinsed with 0.9% sodium chloride (NaCl). The resorption defect was prepared while Cavit™ (3M, Two Harbors, MN, USA) was placed to protect the canal (Figure 25.2) and restored with composite restoration (Figure 25.3). The flap was well irrigated with 0.9% NaCl. A total of five interrupted silk sutures (4-0) were placed (Figure 25.4). A rubber dam (RD) and clamp were placed over tooth #23. Access was completed. Pulpectomy was performed by instrumentation alongside copious irrigation with 0.5% sodium hypochlorite (NaOCl). The canal was dried and medicated with calcium hydroxide (Ca(OH)$_2$; Ultradent, South Jordan, UT, USA). The access cavity was filled

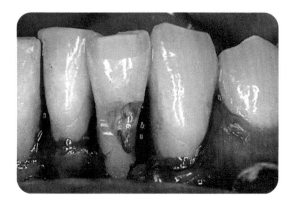

Figure 25.2 The resorption defect was prepared for restoration. Cavit™ was placed to protect the canal space.

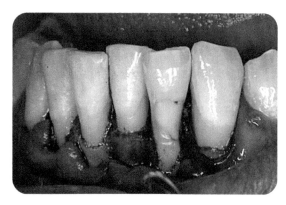

Figure 25.3 The cervical resorptive defect was restored with composite resin.

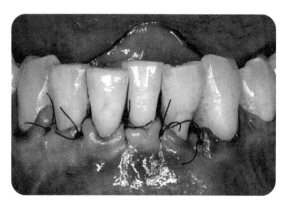

Figure 25.4 The flap was repositioned and interrupted sutures with silk were placed.

with Cavit™. The RD was then removed. Occlusion was adjusted and postoperative instructions (POI) were reviewed including no smoking for at least one week. Pt was advised to use Peridex™ 0.12% (3M, Two Harbors, MN, USA) rinse twice daily for one week and ibuprofen 400 mg every 6–8 hours for pain control.

Day 2 follow-up call: Pt reported very mild postoperative (PO) pain but no medication was required for pain control.

Second visit (1 week): Suture removal visit. Healing of the surgical wound was uneventful. The Pt was made aware that even after comprehensive dental care, the external resorption can return. He was made aware he must have a full mouth series taken to rule out the possibility of resorption involvement in other teeth. An appointment was scheduled for completion of NSRCT.

Third visit (2 months): Continuation of NSRCT for tooth #23. The medical history was reviewed (RMHX). Local anesthesia 54 mg 2% lido/0.027 mg epi (1:100,000) was administered. After RD isolation and access preparation,

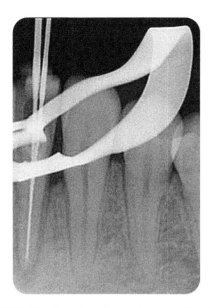

Figure 25.5 Working-length radiograph measuring the length of the canal.

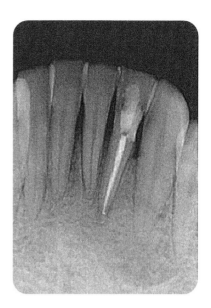

Figure 25.6 Radiograph was taken after obturation of root canal.

buccal (B) and lingual (L) canals, which were joined at the apical 2 mm, were located. A working length was established and confirmed with a radiograph (Figure 25.5). Mechanical instrumentation was performed with .04 taper EndoSequence® rotary files (Brasseler USA, Savannah, GA, USA) using a crown down technique and copious irrigation with 0.5% NaOCl. Canals were dried with paper points. Master cone gutta-percha (GP) points were then placed to length with AH Plus® Root Canal Sealer (Dentsply Sirona, Konstanz, Germany). Canals were filled by System B™ (Kerr, Orange, CA, USA) and back-filled using Calamus® Dual (Dentsply Sirona, Johnson City, TN, USA). Tooth #23 was temporarily filled with Cavit™ and Fuji® IX GP (GC America Inc., Alsip, IL, USA). A PO radiograph was taken (Figure 25.6). PO instructions were reviewed. The Pt was scheduled for a follow-up appointment.

Working length, apical size, and obturation technique

Canal	Working Length	Apical Size	Obturation Material and Techniques
B	21.5 mm	40	GP, AH Plus® sealer, Vertical condensation
L	22.5 mm	40	GP, AH Plus® sealer, Vertical condensation

Postoperative Evaluation

Fourth visit (15-month follow-up): RMHX. Tooth #23 was asymptomatic and non-tender to percussion and palpation. Apex appeared normal in the periapical film (Figure 25.7). The temporary restoration was still in place.

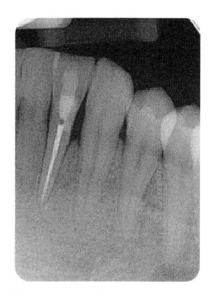

Figure 25.7 Fifteen-month follow-up radiograph shows no sign of periradicular pathosis or recurrence of the resorption.

Gingiva margin was slightly inflamed. Mobility was normal. Pt was advised to schedule a dental hygiene appointment, permanent restoration, and a follow-up.

Fifth visit (2-year follow-up): RMHX. Tooth #23 was asymptomatic. The tooth had been restored with composite core build-up in the access opening by general dentist. Apex appeared normal (Figure 25.8). No resorptive lesion was noted. Mobility was normal. Tooth gingiva margin was slightly inflamed (Figure 25.9). Oral hygiene instruction was given. Satisfactory healing had been achieved.

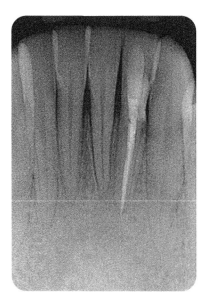

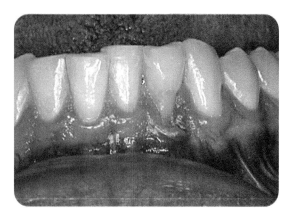

Figure 25.9 Two-year follow-up shows the composite resin restoration was intact with no signs of recurrence of the cervical resorption.

Figure 25.8 Two-year follow-up radiograph shows no evidence of periapical pathosis or extension of the treated resorptive lesion.

Self-Study Questions

A. What are the tooth resorption classifications?

B. What are the etiology of and treatment for internal root resorption?

C. What are the etiology of and treatment for external inflammatory and replacement root resorption?

D. What are the classifications of invasive cervical resorption?

E. What are the treatments for invasive cervical resorption?

Answers to Self-Study Questions

A. Tooth resorptions are classified by Heithersay (2007) into three broad groups:

1. Trauma Induced Tooth Resorption, with subcategories including:
   Surface Resorption
   Transient Apical Internal Resorption
   Pressure Resorption and Orthodontic Resorption
   Replacement Resorption
2. Infection Induced Tooth Resorption, with subcategories including:
   Internal Inflammatory (Infective) Root Resorption
   External Inflammatory Root Resorption
   Communicating Internal-External Inflammatory
      Resorption
3. Hyperplastic Invasive Resorptions with subcategories including:
   Internal replacement (invasive) resorption
   Invasive Coronal Resorption
   Invasive Cervical Resorption

Root resorptions are classified by Fuss, Tsesis & Lin (2003) into five groups:

1. Pulpal Infection Root Resorption
2. Periodontal Infection Root Resorption
3. Orthodontic Pressure Root Resorption
4. Impacted Tooth or Tumor Pressure Root Resorption
5. Ankylotic Root Resorption

Endodontists are often challenged in particular by internal root resorption, external inflammatory root resorption, replacement (ankylotic) root resorption, and invasive cervical resorption.

B. Internal root resorption is due to pulp inflammation or infection (Andreasen 1985; Tronstad 1988; Bakland 1992). The pulp may go through a dynamic change from pulpitis to necrosis. Pulpectomy is performed when pulp is vital. For necrotic pulp, root canal debridement, calcium hydroxide medication, and root canal filling are the treatments.

C. External inflammatory root resorption occurs when pulp becomes necrotic following a traumatic injury. The bacteria and bacterial products in the root canal are the cause and could be exposed to the root surface due to the traumatic damage to cementum (Andreasen 1985; Tronstad 1988; Bakland 1992; Fuss et al. 2003). Inflammatory root resorption is treated by the complete debridement of the root canal and the placement of calcium hydroxide (Tronstad 1988; Heithersay 2007; Komabayashi & Zhu 2012). Root canal filling follows resorption arresting. Replacement resorption may occur due to the death of periodontal ligament cells following replantation of an avulsed tooth. The prognosis is poor. If in a satisfactory position, the tooth can be left in situ and intervention is not needed. In some cases, surgical reposition with root surface Emdogain® treatment may be performed (Filippi, Pohl & von Arx 2006).

D. The etiology of invasive cervical resorption is largely unknown. Invasive cervical resorption is divided by Heithersay (1999) into four classes:

Class 1: A smaller invasive resorptive lesion near the cervical area with shallow penetration into dentine.

Class 2: A well-defined invasive resorptive lesion that has penetrated close to the coronal pulp chamber but shows little or no extension into the radicular dentine.

Class 3: A deeper invasion of dentine by resorbing tissue, not only involving the coronal dentine but also extending at least to the coronal third of the root.

Class 4: A large invasive resorptive process that has extended beyond the coronal third of the root.

E. Non-surgical treatment for invasive cervical resorption includes topical application of 90% aqueous trichloracetic acid to resorptive tissue, curettage, cavity preparation, and glass ionomer cement or composite resin restoration (Heithersay 1999; Fuss *et al.* 2003; Heithersay 2007). Surgical treatment includes flap reflection, curettage, 90% aqueous trichloracetic acid application, cavity preparation, and glass ionomer cement or compos-

ite resin restoration (Heithersay 1999; Fuss *et al.* 2003; Heithersay 2007). Pulpectomy is routinely performed for Class 3 resorption. Class 4 resorption has a poor prognosis and may require tooth extraction.

References

Andreasen, J. O. (1985) External root resorption: Its implication in dental traumatology, paedodontics, periodontics, orthodontics, and endodontics. *International Endodontic Journal* **18**, 109–118.

Bakland, L. K. (1992) Root resorption. *Dental Clinics of North America* **36**, 491–507.

Filippi, A., Pohl, Y. & von Arx, T. (2006) Treatment of replacement resorption by intentional replantation, resection of the ankylosed sites, and Emdogain – results of a 6-year survey. *Dental Traumatology* **22**, 307–311.

Fuss, Z., Tsesis, I. & Lin, S. (2003) Root resorption – diagnosis, classification and treatment choices based on stimulation factors. *Dental Traumatology* **19**, 175–182.

Heithersay, G. S. (1999) Treatment of invasive cervical resorption: An analysis of results using topical application of trichloracetic acid, curettage, and restoration. *Quintessence International* **30**, 96–110.

Heithersay, G. S. (2007) Management of tooth resorption. *Australian Dental Journal* **52** (Suppl. 1), S105–121.

Komabayashi, T. & Zhu, Q. (2012) Internal and external resorption in a lower molar with an associated endodontic-periodontic lesion: A case report. *Australian Endodontic Journal* **38**, 80–84.

Tronstad, L. (1988) Root resorption – etiology, terminology and clinical manifestations. *Endodontics & Dental Traumatology* **4**, 241–252.

INDEX for *Clinical Cases in Endodontics*

Clinical Cases in Endodontics, First Edition. Edited by Takashi Komabayashi.

© 2018 John Wiley & Sons, Inc. Published 2018 by John Wiley & Sons, Inc.

Printed and bound by CPI Group (UK) Ltd, Croydon, CR0 4YY